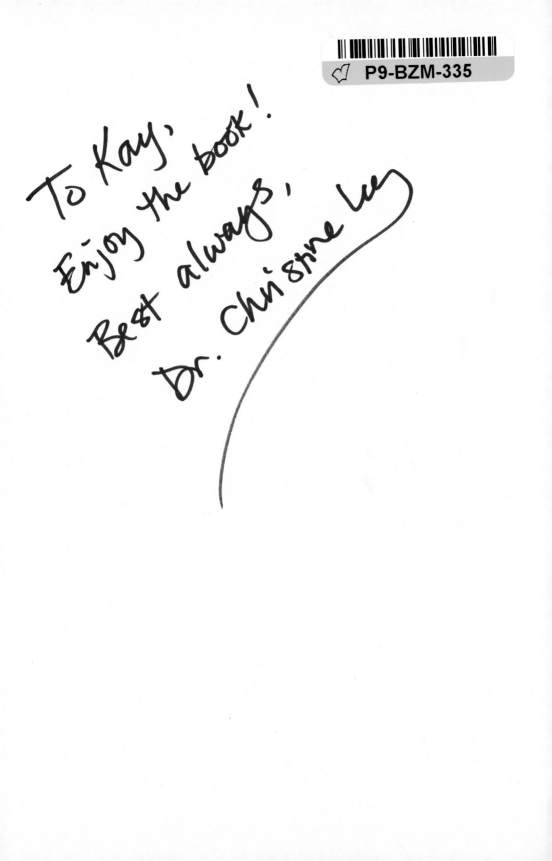

To Kay,
Enjoy the book!
Best always,
Dr. Christine Ley

To you,
Enjoy the book!
Best wishes,
Dr. Chisman

THE
ULTIMATE GUIDE
FOR THE
BEST SKIN EVER:
LASERS

by
M. CHRISTINE LEE, M.D.

Bloomington, IN Milton Keynes, UK

authorHOUSE

AuthorHouse™
1663 Liberty Drive, Suite 200
Bloomington, IN 47403
www.authorhouse.com
Phone: 1-800-839-8640

AuthorHouse™ UK Ltd.
500 Avebury Boulevard
Central Milton Keynes, MK9 2BE
www.authorhouse.co.uk
Phone: 08001974150

This book is a work of non-fiction. Unless otherwise noted, the author and the publisher make no explicit guarantees as to the accuracy of the information contained in this book and in some cases, names of people and places have been altered to protect their privacy.

First published by AuthorHouse 8/25/2006

ISBN: 1-4259-1486-1 (sc)
ISBN: 1-4259-1487-X (dj)

Printed in the United States of America
Bloomington, Indiana

This book is printed on acid-free paper.

This book is dedicated to my loving husband, without whom this book would not be possible, and my family for all their support.

CONTENTS

THE
ULTIMATE GUIDE
FOR THE
BEST SKIN EVER:
LASERS

Chapter 1:

Prologue/Reason for Writing this Book

I SEE PATIENTS EVERYDAY in my Walnut Creek private practice. I love what I do and have a great passion for my specialty. I have been blessed to have the best training and background to allow me to be at the top of my field. Having treated thousands of people during my years of practice, I have a great wealth of experience and knowledge to draw from.

I can only see and treat so many people in a day. I'm not writing this book to get more clientele. I'm already booked out over 3 to 4 months and have people flying in from all over the country and other parts of the world just to have me treat them. If I could invent a tele-porter device so that everyone who wanted to see me could without having constraints due to distance, I still wouldn't be able to see them all. So this book is my way of disseminating the knowledge that I give to my patients daily and make it available for the rest of the world who can't get in to see me. Take this information as knowledge that will empower you to make the right decisions for yourself. I wrote this book so you could have access to the information I know without having to make an appointment to see me. Knowledge is power. My hope is to empower each person who reads this book. I want each person who reads this book to be able to have the same ability that I have when I'm assessing another doctor or practice's legitimacy and ability to provide the quality of services that I would be looking for if I were seeking treatment for a family member or myself.

There are seemingly hundreds (perhaps thousands) of different laser and light devices. Lasers are a big money making business that more and more companies want to get a piece of the pie. And it's a very big pie. In 1998 there were only a handful of legitimate laser companies. Now there are dozens of laser companies that make devices for skin rejuvenation, hair removal, and treatment of vascular and pigmented lesions. However, there are still only a handful of "big" players, companies that are true leaders in the field and develop innovative technology that establish industry standards.

An innovative laser company will invest money in research and development which proves to be fruitful, employ top engineers who have vision and the requisite skills to execute that vision, have the necessary marketing and distribution channels to sell their product, be profitable and reinvest those back in new research and development. They do not sit on their laurels—they know that the industry is highly competitive and the threat of looming new technology that could supplant their own always exists.

Successful innovation can produce a laser that can change the face of medicine and the way physicians treat their patients. It opens the door to treat medical or cosmetic conditions that previously were not possible. When such an invention occurs, many other companies try to emulate and jump on the bandwagon. Suddenly there are dozens of copycats, which may or may not be comparable to the original. There are marketing schemes and advertising gimmicks to try to sway doctors and patients into using their products—claiming their laser is superior to all others.

Good laser companies employ talented engineers and scientists, allocate money for research and development, promote their lasers in an ethical manner, follow health and safety standards, work closely with physicians who have valuable clinical experience, have good marketing and distribution channels, have a strong sales force, and most important of all, produce lasers that work and are safe. Efficacy and safety are equally important. The most effective laser in the world is undesirable if it has a high complication profile.

Laser companies make good investment opportunities but it's important to know which lasers work well. The more established laser companies have superior distribution networks and can provide better maintenance and service. Doctors who use their lasers can have the confidence of knowing that their laser has been clinically tested and proven to be effective and safe. They also should have service contracts guaranteeing that their laser will be repaired within a short period of time if it breaks down or needs a spare part.

I believe that lasers are the number one defense against aging because they can produce natural-appearing changes that are healthy for the skin and they are long lasting. The changes that are achieved are permanent in the sense that they don't "wear off". You can't stop aging, unfortunately, but you can slow it down and reverse some of the damage in order to turn back the clock. Laser treatments can make the skin look 10 to 20 years younger. If you had laser resurfacing done at age 50 and it made you look 40, then in 10 years, you'll be 60 and probably look 50 instead of 60. Compare this to Botox™ and temporary fillers (i.e., Collagen, Cosmoderm®, Restylane®, Perlane®, etc.), which wear off, there are no long-lasting effects, and you go back to looking exactly how you did before.

Because it's so difficult to keep up with the explosion and rapid influx of new information in laser technology and because of all the hype that goes along with it, I saw a need to provide the consumer with a guide to help sort through all the hype and find out what works best for them.

CHAPTER 2:

REVIEW OF LASERS

PEOPLE OFTEN WONDER HOW do lasers work and how do they differ from normal light? Lasers essentially are a more concentrated and focused beam of light and they can vary in the color of light that is used. Different lasers have different functions—some can treat blood vessels and others can destroy hair. Still others can remove wrinkles and scars.

Lasers are essentially a highly focused intense beam of light within a certain wavelength (band of color spectrum). The visible and invisible light spectrum is composed of the following colors: infrared, red, orange, yellow, green, blue, indigo, violet, and ultraviolet. The cornerstone of laser physics is the theory of selective photothermolysis which was first described by Dr. R. Rox Anderson and Dr. John Parrish in 1983.[1] They theorized that an object containing a chromophore (a light absorbing molecule such as oxyhemoglobin or melanin—oxyhemoglobin makes red blood cells red, and melanin is the brown pigment in skin) can be selectively targeted for destruction if it is exposed to a wavelength of light that is preferentially absorbed by that chromophore and at an exposure time that is equal to or less than the object's thermal relaxation time. Thermal relaxation time is the time required for an object to lose half of its thermal energy.

Lasers by definition are a collimated high intensity focused beam of light within a specific wavelength. Collimated means that the light beam rays are parallel and focused instead of being scattered. Think of a marching band all wearing the same uniforms marching in one direction compared to a crowd of people wearing all different clothes that are milling around in no order. The marching band is like the collimated beam of light. The crowd of people is like normal light, which is diffuse and scattered.

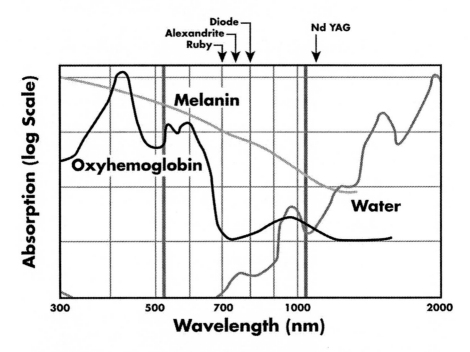

Lasers can be very effective for targeting specific objects such as hair, vascular and pigmented lesions. Some lasers are best absorbed by water and are used for ablation or vaporation of the skin. This is called laser resurfacing, which causes a superficial burn or injury to the skin, which causes the skin to slough off and leave behind brand new smoother skin, similar to the pink skin of a baby's bottom. These ablative lasers (i.e., carbon dioxide (CO_2), Erbium:YAG) are the gold standards for removing wrinkles and are also widely used for treating textural irregularities of the skin and also for acne scarring.

Some lasers are ideally absorbed by oxyhemoglobin, the pigment contained within red blood cells that give them their red color. These lasers include argon, holmium, pulsed dye, and KTP (potassium titanyl phosphate) lasers. Other lasers are ideally suited for treating pigmented lesions due to their high specificity for melanin. These include the ruby, alexandrite, Q-switched Nd:YAG, and KTP lasers.

Since 1999, the noninvasive or nonablative lasers have become the dominant lasers on the market due to their ability to stimulate collagen and improve skin tone and texture without causing injury to the skin. They were originally touted to be the better alternative to the CO2 laser for removing wrinkles without the downtime and complications associated with the CO2. The problem with these lasers has been that the results have not been as impressive. It turns out that in order to adequately remove wrinkles, some injury needs to take place in order to effectively erase the wrinkle. Ablative resurfacing with the CO2 or Erbium:YAG lasers cause an injury to the skin, which physically re-moves the top layer of damaged skin and allows new undamaged skin to take its place. The skin wrinkles because of aging caused by sun damage and the person's own biological aging mechanism. Everyone is pre-programmed genetically to age at a certain rate—this is called biological aging. You can then drastically speed up the aging clock by having constant exposure to the sun and also by unhealthy habits such as smoking and using certain illicit drugs. The key to younger looking skin is to remove the outermost damaged layer of skin.

Noninvasive lasers by definition do not cause injury to the outer layer of skin. They work by using thermal (heat) energy to cause a thermal injury to the underlying skin, which stimulates a cascade of re-sponses within the skin cells to produce new collagen. The principles of nonablative resurfacing are based on a theory of collagen remodeling, which involve heating of cells (called fibroblasts), which then release chemicals in response to the heat injury to produce new collagen. The new collagen then causes a plumping effect of the skin, which trans-lates into more elastic and better skin tone. This can visibly be seen as a healthier color to the skin, tighter pores, smoother texture, and reduced wrinkles. Many people describe their skin as having a "radiant glow" after these treatments. All sounds great unless you have deeper wrinkles. Then the improvement can be negligible and the patient is left wanting for more. And that more is inevitably using the CO2 or Erbium laser for invasive or ablative resurfacing.

A variety of lasers are used for removing tattoos. Different colors of tattoos need to be treated by different laser wavelengths, which are specific for absorption by that specific color. Someone with a multicolored tattoo may need 3 or 4 different lasers to get optimal clearance.

Other lasers are used for leg vein treatments. The difficulty in treating leg veins is that there are all sorts of different leg veins. Some veins are red or purple or blue in color. They also vary in terms of depth in the skin and also by size or diameter of the vessel. There are varicose veins, which are the big ropey or snakelike large veins, which protrude. Then there are smaller spider veins that can vary in color (red, purple, or blue) and even smaller telangiectasias or broken capillaries. Some veins appear like permanent bruises which is called telangiectactic matting (these are ultra fine tiny broken capillaries which form a network or cluster which appear as a large bruise on the leg).

The laser selected for proper treatment depends on the color, size, diameter, and depth of the vein. Some lasers will work on the red veins (which contain oxyhemoglobin) and others work on blue veins (which contain **de**oxygenated hemoglobin so it no longer has the red pigment) and purple veins (which contain a combination of oxygenated and deoxygenated hemoglobin).

Another important factor that needs to be taken in consideration when choosing the appropriate laser is the patient's skin type. Certain lasers are safe for all skin types and others are more dangerous for use on darker or tan skin.

There is a whole other category of devices that are not true lasers but are light devices. These are broad-spectrum lights that have wavelengths that cover a wide spectrum of colors instead of being specific for one color wavelength. Also, they're diffuse and scattered instead of being collimated, high intensity, and focused as lasers are. They are much more like the crowd of people instead of the marching band.

Light devices are not as specific for targeting objects due to the nonspecificity of the light source. In general, they are less specific and therefore less effective than lasers for treating various targets. The most common light source is the intense pulsed light (IPL) also commonly known as the "FotoFacial." IPL can be used to treat hair, vascular and pigmented lesions. It is used in a process called photorejuvenation that removes sun damage. "Photo" refers to sun damaged skin. Photorejuvenation can be accomplished with either lasers or IPL.

The advantage of IPL devices over lasers is that in general they are less expensive than lasers, they have larger spot sizes (the size of the handpiece) which results in faster treatments, and they are rather broad in their applications (the same device can be used to remove hair, treat vascular and pigmented lesions, treat rosacea, perform photorejuvenation, and treat acne). The disadvantage is that IPL devices are usually less effective than lasers due to their lower specificity and lower energies, and can be more problematic in treating darker or tan skin. The larger spot sizes are cumbersome and difficult to use in treating more contoured surfaces such as the eye or nose area. Imagine trying to fit a rectangular block that measures 1 x 1 cm into the groove around the nostrils to treat some blood vessels. Can't do it with the IPL device. Also, it's not possible to treat lesions located around the eye due to the large spot size. These areas are much more suited to the lasers which have smaller spot sizes (1-2 mm) that can fit anywhere no matter how small or tight the crevice. So the IPL is more desirable for large flat surface areas whereas lasers have more flexibility to treat all different shaped surfaces.

Another category of devices involves radiofrequency. These appeared in 2000 to 2001—the first monopolar radiofrequency device is called the ThermaCool by Thermage (Hayward, CA). It has been nicknamed the nonablative or nonsurgical radiofrequency lift. It uses an electrical source or radiowave to thermally heat the deeper layers of skin to promote collagen remodeling and cause skin tightening and contraction.

Another company called Syneron (Israel) utilizes bipolar radiofrequency coupled with optical light (IPL source). They make a device which uses a different type of radiofrequency that does not penetrate as deeply as the monopolar radiofrequency device so it does not cause the same level of skin tightening but it has been used for hair removal, photorejuvenation, and nonablative resurfacing. Its principles are based on using less light energy by combining it with electrical energy so that it's supposed to make the treatments more safe and effective than IPL alone. It is important not to get this confused with the Thermage device.

A new form of infrared light with a higher intensity source of light than normal IPL devices came out recently called the Titan by Cutera (Brisbane, CA). It is trying to compete with the Thermage device as a skin tightening procedure. It works by delivering a pulse of light that penetrates deeper than normal IPL devices so it also can result in more effective collagen remodeling and skin tightening and contraction. I performed a study comparing the Thermage and Titan devices and presented this study at the American Society for Dermatologic Surgery annual meeting in Atlanta, October 2005.

I had patients separated into 3 separate groups: (1) Patients receiving half-face treatment with Thermage compared to half-face control (without any treatment), (2) Patients receiving half-face treatment with Titan compared to half-face control, (3) Patients receiving half-face treatment with Thermage (one treatment) compared to half-face with Titan (1 to 3 treatments). The reason I had to increase the number of treatments on the Titan side was because it became apparent early on during the study that some of the patients receiving only one Titan treatment were not having any results, so I had to increase the number of treatments with Titan in order to determine if increasing the number of treatments would help improve treatment efficacy. In the end, I concluded that both treatments are effective for skin tightening but that the Titan side required more treatments to produce the same results as one Thermage treatment. In general, it takes about 2 or 3 Titan treatments to give the results of one Thermage treatment. Another disadvantage with the Titan device is that it takes twice as long to complete a full-face treatment compared to the Thermage device. An advantage of the Titan is that it is less painful than the original Thermage device. (Pain used to be an issue for the Thermage procedure. However, Thermage developed a new tip in late 2005 which has made pain a nonissue and still provides the same results). In order to tolerate either treatment, the settings need to be turned down lower and in order to compensate for lower energy, the physician needs to do more "passes" (number of times going over the face) to optimize results. Doing more passes requires more time.

Another problem with the Titan device which is more relevant for the operator of the device and less so for the patient, is that the Titan handpiece is heavy and awkward and difficult to use and see while treating. In comparison, the Thermage handpiece is lighter with less strain on the operator's hand and also has better visibility for the operator to see where they are treating.

A new class of devices called LED (light emitting diode) has been popular in the spa market. Mostly because they're very low energy and not capable of causing injury to the skin so they're considered safer, but they also have negligible effects. I have seen before and after photos demonstrating amazing results but when trying these devices in real life, I have not been able to detect any visible improvements. If the LED devices are used with a light activated chemical called 5-aminolevulinic acid (5-ALA), there can be some results seen that are similar to a chemical peel. However, 5-ALA can be activated with any light, laser, or LED source, so it's not necessary to buy an LED device just to activate 5-ALA. In fact, 5-ALA can be activated by just sitting under a fluorescent light or by exposure to sunlight. A blue light manufactured by DUSA called the BLU-U is a far less costly means of activating 5-ALA than using light, laser, or LED sources.

Many things can stimulate collagen production including mechanical (microdermabrasion), chemical (peels containing trichloroacetic acid, glycolic acid, or other acids), or heat (light, laser, radiofrequency, LED). Even slapping the face can cause collagen stimulation. The big question is how much collagen production is required in order to see substantial reduction of wrinkles. Being able to detect new collagen formation histologically by examining a piece of skin underneath the microscope is one thing, being able to see visible wrinkle reduction and smoothing or tightening of the face is another. There was a device called Primos which was being marketed by Johnson & Johnson which was a high tech device used to analyze the amount of collagen that was being produced under the skin—it would produce a computer generated topographic map. The problem with this device is that it had no applicable use. In real life, if results cannot be seen from a simple before and after photograph, it doesn't matter what the Primos system can show you.

Trying to decide which device (light, laser, or radiofrequency) will give you the best results is a bewildering process. I have developed a comparison chart to help with the decision making process. The devices are categorized based on the problem or condition (i.e.: rosacea, sun damage, leg veins, hair removal, etc.) being treated. They are given a grade (A thru F) in order to rank their effectiveness and provide a reference for comparison. Most of the most common lasers are listed but it is by no means a complete list. There are so many lasers, some produced by new start-up laser companies which may not have been tested yet, that it is not possible to have a complete listing and ranking of every laser brand available. My goal is to help the consumer be able to categorize lasers based on type and be able to know which types of lasers are best to treat which kinds of conditions.

Many laser companies make claims that their laser treats many conditions ranging from acne, rosacea, sun damage, photorejuvenation, vascular and pigmented lesions, wrinkles, hair removal, tattoo removal, skin tightening, to acne scarring, stretchmarks, leg veins, surgical scars, and textural irregularities. One laser may receive an A for laser hair removal but a C for rosacea. I have given ratings to lasers that claim to treat certain conditions. Some lasers when used by themselves may only have a C rating but when combined with a laser with a B rating for a certain condition, may actually be able to achieve B+ or better results when the 2 lasers are combined together to achieve a synergistic result. Two B+ lasers combined together might give "A" level results for a certain condition.

Rosacea is a chronic skin condition that causes individuals to flush or blush easily. It can also be associated with acne breakouts, large pores, and sebaceous prominence (which appear as raised bumps on the face and also cause the nose to become enlarged—W.C. Fields is the classic example). The constant flushing condition causes blood vessels or capillaries to dilate and appear enlarged. The lasers that best treat this condition are specific for oxyhemoglobin and target blood vessels. Some patients with rosacea also get enlarged blue and purple blood vessels—these are best treated by long-pulsed Nd:YAG (infrared) lasers. Many conditions are best treated when combining multiple modalities. In many rosacea patients, I combine the KTP and Nd:YAG lasers with IPL. KTP is the best laser wavelength to treat individual red blood vessels. Nd:YAG laser is best for blue and purple vessels. IPL is effective for background blush and since it utilizes a larger handpiece, allows me to perform more passes on the face to save time so then I can hone in on individual blood vessels with the KTP and perform fewer passes over the whole face with the KTP (since it takes longer than IPL).

Many lasers companies are developing laser systems that contain several lasers within one unit—in these multiple laser systems, I have given each separate laser module within that system an individual rating. Examples of laser systems containing multiple lasers are the Gemini (Laserscope), Lumenis One (Lumenis), Profile (Sciton), CoolGlide XEO (Cutera), Genesis Plus (Cutera).

Grading system used for comparison charts: A through F. A+ is the highest rating, F- is the lowest rating.

Top Lasers for Rosacea:

1. 532 nm/KTP (green) laser
   Brand/Company: Gemini/Laserscope (A+), Aura/Laserscope (A)

2. 585 or 595 nm/Pulsed dye (yellow) laser
   Vbeam/Candela (B+)

3. Intense Pulsed Light
   Aurora/Syneron (B-), Quantum/Lumenis (B-), EsteLux/Palomar (B-)

Comparison Chart for Rosacea

Class or type of laser	Wavelength/Color	Brand Name/Company	Grade
Pulsed dye laser	595 nm/yellow	Vbeam/Candela	B+
Pulsed dye laser	585 nm/yellow	Cbeam/Candela	B
Pulsed dye laser	585 nm/yellow	Photogenica/Cynosure	B
Pulsed dye laser	585-595 nm/yellow	Sclerolase/Candela	B+
KTP and	532 nm/green &	Gemini/Laserscope	A+
Nd:YAG	1064 nm/infrared		C

KTP	532 nm/green	Aura/Laserscope	A
KTP	532 nm/green	Diolite/Iridex	B+
KTP	532 nm/green	VariLite/Iridex	B+
KTP	532 nm/green	Versapulse/Lumenis	A-
Intense Pulsed Light	400-1400 nm/IPL	StarLux/Palomar	B-
Intense Pulsed Light	400-1400 nm/IPL	MediLux/Palomar	B-
Intense Pulsed Light	400-1400 nm/IPL	EsteLux/Palomar	B-
Intense Pulsed Light	560-1200 nm/IPL	IPL Quantum SR/ Lumenis	B-
Intense Pulsed Light	515-1200 nm/IPL	VascuLight Elite/ Lumenis	B-
Intense Pulsed Light	515-1200 nm/IPL	Lumenis One/Lumenis	B-
Intense Pulsed Light	600-850 nm/IPL	CoolGlide XEO/Cutera	B-
Intense Pulsed Light	560 nm/IPL	560LP/Cutera	B-
Intense Pulsed Light	500-610 nm/IPL	Clareon VR/Novalis	B-
Intense Pulsed Light	520-1200 nm/IPL	Solarus VR/Novalis	B-
Pulsed Light + Radiofrequency	580-980 nm/IPL	Aurora SR/Syneron	B-
Light Heat Energy	400-1200 nm/IPL	SkinStation/Radiancy	B-
Nd:YAG	1064 nm/infrared	CoolGlide Excel/Cutera	D-
Nd:YAG	1064 nm/infrared	Lyra/Laserscope	C

Even though the pulsed dye laser is well absorbed by oxyhemoglobin, there are some other variables that gave this laser a B+ when compared to some KTP systems. Other factors to consider other than wavelength are type of cooling, spot size, and depth of penetration. Different forms of cooling are used to make treatments less painful and safer. Types of cooling include contact cooling (using a sapphire or glass window with a cold water supply continuously surrounding the glass to chill the glass to a temperature of 5° C. The Candela lasers (Vbeam and Cbeam) have cryogen cooling (a spray of cold liquid nitrogen mist to chill the skin prior to the laser beam firing). Other systems use a cold blast of air blowing over the skin. Less sophisticated systems do not have a built-in cooler. In addition to using built-in cooling systems, a chilled lubricant (ultrasound gel, KY jelly, Aloe Vera) is applied to the skin to protect it.

I believe that continuous contact cooling is the superior method to cool the skin. There are certain lasers that utilize that form of cooling and I think that makes these lasers safer. The problem with using cryogen cooling (the liquid nitrogen spray) is that there can be over freezing of the skin which can cause a "cryogen burn" which in certain skin types (especially darker or ethnic skin) can result in hyperpigmentation (brown-red discolorations), hypopigmentation (loss of pigment), or scarring.

The Gemini laser is a combination of 2 different lasers in one box: the 532 nm/KTP and the 1064 nm/Nd:YAG. It is the best laser for vascular and pigmented lesions for several reasons: (1) It utilizes contact cooling, (2) The clear glass handpiece is easy to visualize the lesions being treated, (3) The Gemini has a variable spot size that can be adjusted from 1 to 10 mm which allows it to treat lesions of all different sizes and penetrates to different levels beneath the skin. Some other systems (i.e., Diolite) have a smaller spot size (up to 1.4 mm), which makes it less effective in treating certain larger blood vessels and vessels that are located deeper. The Diolite also does not have contact cooling. So not all KTP lasers are alike. Same with all other similar laser and light devices—one IPL may be superior to another because of individual characteristics.

The Vbeam is effective at treating fine superficial broken blood vessels but less effective at treating larger and deeper blood vessels. This has to do with the variations in spot size, energy levels, and type of cooling being used. Some vessels may require multiple repeat passes in order to shut them down. But when using a laser with cryogen spray cooling, there may be too much freezing of the skin that would prevent doing multiple passes. This is why doing multiple passes with a laser that uses contact cooling is more effective—one does not have to worry that going over the same lesion several times would result in a freeze burn.

The Versapulse was a very good laser but has unfortunately been discontinued and no longer manufactured by Lumenis. Doctors who own this system may have difficulty getting parts for this laser.

IPL devices are very effective for treating the blushing associated with rosacea but not as effective for treating individual blood vessels, especially those around the nose. The IPL systems that have built-in cooling received a higher grade because of safety issues. All IPL devices (except the Cutera 560LP) need to be used with a cooling gel.

The long-pulsed Nd:YAG lasers (Lyra, CoolGlide) received lower ratings for rosacea because this wavelength is not well-absorbed by oxy-hemoglobin. However, lasers with this wavelength are ideally suited for treating blue veins that contain deoxygenated hemoglobin. Some patients with rosacea need a combination of both a visible green or yellow wavelength (pulsed dye laser, KTP) to treat the red vessels and a long-pulsed Nd:YAG laser (Lyra, CoolGlide) to treat the blue vessels. If a long-pulsed Nd:YAG laser were combined with a KTP laser, then it would provide A+ results (see Gemini laser which is a combination of KTP and Nd:YAG laser).

Top Lasers for Red Blood Vessels:

1. 532 nm/KTP (green) laser
   Brand/Company: Gemini/Laserscope (A+), Aura/Laserscope (A+), Diolite/Iridex (B+)

2. 585 nm/Pulsed dye (yellow) laser
   Vbeam/Candela (B+)

3. Intense Pulsed Light
   Acutip/Cutera (B+), Aurora/Syneron (B-), Quantum/Lumenis (B-), EsteLux/Palomar (B-)

Comparison Chart for Red Blood Vessels

Class or Type of Laser	Wavelength/Color	Brand Name/Company	Grade
Pulsed dye laser	595 nm/yellow	Vbeam/Candela	B+
Pulsed dye laser	585 nm/yellow	Cbeam/Candela	B
Pulsed dye laser	585 nm/yellow	Photogenica/Cynosure	B
Pulsed dye laser	585-595 nm/yellow	Sclerolase/Candela	B+
KTP and	532 nm/green &	Gemini/Laserscope	A+
Nd:YAG	1064 nm/infrared		C

KTP	532 nm/green	Aura/Laserscope	A+
KTP	532 nm/green	Diolite/Iridex	B+
KTP and Diode	532 nm/green & 940 nm	VariLite/Iridex	B+ D
KTP	532 nm/green	Versapulse/Lumenis	A
Intense Pulsed Light and Nd:YAG laser	400-1400 nm/IPL & 1064 nm	StarLux/Palomar	B- D
Intense Pulsed Light	400-1400 nm/IPL	MediLux/Palomar	B-
Intense Pulsed Light	400-1400 nm/IPL	EsteLux/Palomar	B-
Intense Pulsed Light	560-1200 nm/IPL	IPL Quantum SR/ Lumenis	B-
Intense Pulsed Light	515-1200 nm/IPL	VascuLight Elite/Lumenis	B-
Intense Pulsed Light	515-1200 nm/IPL	Lumenis One/Lumenis	B-
Intense Pulsed Light	600-850 nm/IPL	CoolGlide XEO/Cutera	B-
Intense Pulsed Light	560 nm/IPL	560LP/Cutera	B-
Intense Pulsed Light	535 nm/IPL	Acutip/Cutera	B+
Intense Pulsed Light	500-610 nm/IPL	Clareon VR/Novalis	B-
Intense Pulsed Light	520-1200 nm/IPL	Solarus VR/Novalis	B-
Pulsed Light + Radiofrequency	580-980 nm/IPL	Aurora SR/Syneron	B-
Diode + Radiofrequency	900 nm	Polaris Vascular/Syneron	D-
Light Heat Energy	400-1200 nm/IPL	SkinStation/Radiancy	C
Nd:YAG	1064 nm/infrared	CoolGlide Excel/Cutera	D-
Nd:YAG	1064 nm/infrared	CoolGlide Vantage/Cutera	D-
Intense Pulsed Light & Nd:YAG	600-850 nm/IPL & 1064 nm/infrared	CoolGlide XEO/Cutera	B- D-
Nd:YAG	1064 nm/infrared	Lyra/Laserscope	C
Nd:YAG	1064 nm/infrared	Varia/CoolTouch	D-
Nd:YAG	1064 nm/infrared	Profile/Sciton	D-
Nd:YAG	1064 nm/infrared	VascuLight Elite/Lumenis	D-
Intense Pulsed Light & Nd:YAG	560-1200 nm/IPL &1064 nm/infrared	IPL Quantum DL/ Lumenis	B- D-
Nd:YAG	1064 nm/infrared	GentleYAG/Candela	D-
Diode	800 nm	LightSheer/Lumenis	D-

The reason the Lyra laser received a higher rating for individual red vessels than the CoolGlide even though they're both Nd:YAG lasers is because the Lyra has a smaller spot size of 1.5 mm that allows higher energies to be delivered without burning the skin and that helps to compensate for the lower levels of absorption of this wavelength by oxyhemoglobin. The CoolGlide has a larger spot size of 3 mm or greater and is not able to concentrate the higher levels of energy needed to destroy red blood vessels without burning the skin. The Lyra also utilizes continuous contact cooling which provides better cooling of the skin than the CoolGlide which utilizes a copper metal plate that does not directly and continuously cool the skin while the laser beam is firing.

Top Lasers for Blue Blood Vessels:

1. Long-pulsed 1064 nm/Nd:YAG (infrared) laser
   Brand/Company: Lyra/Laserscope (A+), Gemini/Laserscope (A+)*

2. Long-pulsed 1064 nm/Nd:YAG (infrared) laser
   CoolGlide/Cutera (A-), Profile/Sciton (B+), VascuLight/ Lumenis (B+)*

3. 900 nm/Diode + Bipolar radiofrequency laser
   Polaris Vascular/Syneron (B)

Note: Even though rankings 1 and 2 are the same "type" of lasers, there's enough individual variation to warrant a higher ranking for the Laserscope lasers.

Comparison Chart for Blue Blood Vessels

Class or Type of Laser	Wavelength/Color	Brand Name/Company	Grade
Pulsed dye laser	595 nm/yellow	Vbeam/Candela	D
Pulsed dye laser	585 nm/yellow	Cbeam/Candela	D
Pulsed dye laser	585 nm/yellow	Photogenica/Cynosure	D

Pulsed dye laser	585-595 nm/yellow	Sclerolase/Candela	D
KTP and	532 nm/green &	Gemini/Laserscope	C
Nd:YAG	1064 nm/infrared		A+
KTP	532 nm/green	Aura/Laserscope	C
KTP	532 nm/green	Diolite/Iridex	D+
KTP and Diode	532 nm/green &	VariLite/Iridex	D+
	940 nm/infrared		B-
KTP	532 nm/green	Versapulse/Lumenis	C
Intense Pulsed Light	400-1400 nm/IPL	StarLux/Palomar	D
and infrared laser	& 1064 nm/infrared		B+
Intense Pulsed Light	400-1400 nm/IPL	MediLux/Palomar	D
Intense Pulsed Light	400-1400 nm/IPL	EsteLux/Palomar	D
Intense Pulsed Light	560 nm/IPL	560LP/Cutera	F
Intense Pulsed Light	500-610 nm/IPL	Clareon VR/Novalis	F
Intense Pulsed Light	520-1200 nm/IPL	Solarus VR/Novalis	D
Pulsed Light +	580-980 nm/IPL	Aurora SR/Syneron	D-
Radiofrequency			
Diode + Radiofrequency	900 nm	Polaris Vascular/Syneron	B
Light Heat Energy	400-1200 nm/IPL	SkinStation/Radiancy	D
Nd:YAG	1064 nm/infrared	CoolGlide Excel/Cutera	A-
Nd:YAG	1064 nm/infrared	CoolGlide Vantage/ Cutera	A-
Nd:YAG & IPL	1064 nm/infrared	CoolGlide XEO/Cutera	A-
	& 600-850 nm/IPL		D
Nd:YAG	1064 nm/infrared	Lyra/Laserscope	A+
Nd:YAG	1064 nm/infrared	Varia/CoolTouch	B+
Nd:YAG	1064 nm/infrared	Profile/Sciton	B+
Nd:YAG	1064 nm/infrared	VascuLight Elite/ Lumenis	B+
Intense Pulsed Light	560-1200 nm/IPL	IPL Quantum DL/	D
+ Nd:YAG	+1064 nm/infrared	Lumenis	B+
Nd:YAG	1064 nm/infrared	GentleYAG/Candela	B+
Diode	800 nm	LightSheer/Lumenis	C

Top Lasers for Red, Blue, and Purple Blood Vessels:

1. Long-pulsed 1064 nm/Nd:YAG (infrared) laser
   Brand/Company: Lyra/Laserscope (A+), Gemini/Laserscope (A+)

2. Long-pulsed 1064 nm/Nd:YAG (infrared) laser
   CoolGlide/Cutera (A-), Profile/Sciton (B+), VascuLight/Lumenis (B+)

3. 900 nm/Diode + Bipolar radiofrequency laser
   Polaris Vascular/Syneron (B)

4. 940 nm/Diode + 532 nm/KTP (green) laser
   VariLite/Iridex (B-)

Comparison Chart for Leg Veins (Red, blue and purple vessels)

Class or Type of Laser	Wavelength/Color	Brand Name/Company	Grade
Pulsed dye laser	595 nm/yellow	Vbeam/Candela	D
Pulsed dye laser	585 nm/yellow	Cbeam/Candela	D
Pulsed dye laser	585 nm/yellow	Photogenica/Cynosure	D
Pulsed dye laser	585-595 nm/yellow	Sclerolase/Candela	D
KTP and Nd:YAG	532 nm/green & 1064 nm/infrared	Gemini/Laserscope	A+
KTP	532 nm/green	Aura/Laserscope	C
KTP	532 nm/green	Diolite/Iridex	D+
KTP and Diode	532 nm/green & 940 nm/infrared	VariLite/Iridex	B-
KTP	532 nm/green	Versapulse/Lumenis	C
Intense Pulsed Light and infrared laser	400-1400 nm/IPL & 1064 nm/infrared	StarLux/Palomar	C
Intense Pulsed Light	400-1400 nm/IPL	MediLux/Palomar	D+

Intense Pulsed Light	400-1400 nm/IPL	EsteLux/Palomar	D+
Intense Pulsed Light & Nd:YAG & diode	515-1200 nm/IPL 1064 & 800 nm	Lumenis One/Lumenis	A-
Nd:YAG	1064 nm/infrared	VascuLight Elite/Lumenis	B+
Intense Pulsed Light + Nd:YAG	560-1200 nm/IPL +1064 nm/infrared	IPL Quantum DL/ Lumenis	D+ B+
Intense Pulsed Light	560 nm/IPL	560LP/Cutera	F
Intense Pulsed Light	500-610 nm/IPL	Clareon VR/Novalis	F
Intense Pulsed Light	520-1200 nm/IPL	Solarus VR/Novalis	D-
Pulsed Light + Radiofrequency	580-980 nm/IPL	Aurora SR/Syneron	D-
Diode + Radiofrequency	900 nm	Polaris Vascular/Syneron	B
Light Heat Energy	400-1200 nm/IPL	SkinStation/Radiancy	F
Nd:YAG	1064 nm/infrared	CoolGlide Excel/Cutera	A-
Nd:YAG	1064 nm/infrared	CoolGlide Vantage/Cutera	A-
Nd:YAG & IPL	1064 nm/infrared & 600-850 nm/IPL	CoolGlide XEO/Cutera	A-
Nd:YAG	1064 nm/infrared	Lyra/Laserscope	A+
Nd:YAG	1064 nm/infrared	Varia/CoolTouch	B+
Nd:YAG	1064 nm/infrared	Profile/Sciton	B+
Nd:YAG	1064 nm/infrared	VascuLight Elite/Lumenis	B+
Nd:YAG	1064 nm/infrared	GentleYAG/Candela	B+
Diode	800 nm	LightSheer/Lumenis	C-

Treating leg veins are tricky. Leg veins come in all different colors, sizes, and depth of location in the skin. Some veins are red, very fine, and located superficially near the surface of the skin. Other vessels may be blue and large in diameter and located rather deep below the skin surface. The Lyra laser received the highest rating because it has the highest capability in treating the greatest range of vessels. One of the problems with treating red vessels on the leg with either the KTP or pulsed dye lasers even though they can specifically target oxyhemoglobin is that there is some interference with the patient's own pigment and since the skin on the legs is thicker than facial skin to begin with, higher amounts of energy need to be applied to destroy red veins on the legs. Due to some interference and absorption by the patient's own melanin and the higher energies needed to adequately treat leg veins, there is greater risk of blistering, burning, and loss of pigment if the KTP or pulsed dye lasers are used on leg veins. The problem with most Nd:YAG lasers is that even if they're safer and have greater depth of penetration which allows this wavelength to better penetrate the thicker leg skin, the Nd:YAG wavelength is not specific for oxyhemoglobin, thus being ineffective on red vessels. The Nd:YAG is ideal for treating blue vessels.

In order to treat red and purple vessels adequately without burning the skin, there needs to be an incredibly high amount of energy delivered through a very small spot size so that it is concentrated enough to destroy the red vessel which is not well-absorbed by the infrared/Nd:YAG wavelength. Proper cooling is required to avoid burning the skin. The Lyra satisfies all these criteria. The other Nd:YAG lasers have larger spot sizes and do not have continuous contact cooling so it's not possible to concentrate such a high energy level without possibly burning the skin when treating red vessels on the legs. If a wavelength does not penetrate deep enough in the skin due to either inadequate spot size or inadequate amounts of energy or improper wavelength, then the heat just stays on the surface of the skin and may burn the skin instead of destroying the target. Without adequate cooling, the risk of this occurring is even greater.

The CoolGlide utilizes a copper metal plate to chill the skin which does not cool the treatment area as uniformly as the sapphire contact cooling window that is used in the Lyra laser.

Pigmentation is a very broad category. It can encompass individual brown spots, or freckles, or large brown patches such as melasma. Melasma, also known as the "mask of pregnancy," is a condition that women may develop during pregnancy or while on hormonal supplements. It is a difficult condition to treat if the patient can't get off the hormones. If the pigmentation is solely caused by sun damage, the treatments are much more effective. As you will see, the concept of photorejuvenation evolves around lasers that help to remove pigmented and vascular lesions that are caused by sun damage.

Top Lasers for Pigmentation:

1. 532 nm/KTP (green) laser
    Brand/Company: Aura/Laserscope (A+), Gemini/Laserscope (A+), Diolite/Iridex (A+)

2. Q-switched 532 nm/KTP (green) laser
    Q-YAG 5/Palomar (A), MedLite/HOYA (A)

3. Carbon dioxide (CO2) laser
    Encore/Lumenis (A-), Ultrapulse/Lumenis (A-)

4. Erbium:YAG laser
    Venus/Laserscope (A-), Profile Contour/Sciton (A-)

5. Intense Pulsed Light:
    Acutip/Cutera (A-), 560LP/Cutera (B+), XEO/Cutera (B), EsteLux/Palomar (B), Quantum/Lumenis (B)

Comparison Chart for Pigmentation

Class or Type of Laser	Wavelength/Color	Brand Name/Company	Grade
Pulsed dye laser	595 nm/yellow	Vbeam/Candela	C
Pulsed dye laser	585 nm/yellow	Cbeam/Candela	C
Pulsed dye laser	585 nm/yellow	Photogenica/Cynosure	C
Pulsed dye laser	585-595 nm/yellow	Sclerolase/Candela	C
Pulsed dye laser	585 nm/yellow	NLite/ICN	D
Intense Pulse Light &	500-950 nm/IPL	Cynergy 3/Cynosure	B
Nd:YAG &	& 1064 nm/infrared		F
Pulsed dye laser	& 595 nm/yellow		C
KTP and	532 nm/green &	Gemini/Laserscope	A+
Nd:YAG	1064 nm/infrared		F
KTP	532 nm/green	Aura/Laserscope	A+
KTP	532 nm/green	Diolite/Iridex	A+
KTP and	532 nm/green &	VariLite/Iridex	A+
Diode	940 nm		F
KTP	532 nm/green	Versapulse/Lumenis	A+

Intense Pulsed Light	400-1400 nm/IPL	StarLux/Palomar	B
and Nd:YAG laser	& 1064 nm		F
Intense Pulsed Light	400-1400 nm/IPL	MediLux/Palomar	B
Intense Pulsed Light	400-1400 nm/IPL	EsteLux/Palomar	B
Intense Pulsed Light	560-1200 nm/IPL	IPL Quantum SR/ Lumenis	B
Intense Pulsed Light	515-1200 nm/IPL	VascuLight Elite/ Lumenis	B
Intense Pulsed Light	515-1200 nm/IPL	Lumenis One/Lumenis	B
Intense Pulsed Light	600-850 nm/IPL	CoolGlide XEO/Cutera	B
Intense Pulsed Light	560 nm/IPL	560LP/Cutera	B+
Intense Pulsed Light	535 nm/IPL	Acutip/Cutera	A-
Intense Pulsed Light	500-610 nm/IPL	Clareon VR/Novalis	B
Intense Pulsed Light	520-1200 nm/IPL	Solarus VR/Novalis	B
Pulsed Light + Radiofrequency	580-980 nm/IPL	Aurora SR/Syneron	B
Diode + Radiofrequency	900 nm	Polaris Vascular/Syneron	F
Light Heat Energy	400-1200 nm/IPL	SkinStation/Radiancy	B
Nd:YAG	1064 nm/infrared	CoolGlide Excel/Cutera	F
Nd:YAG	1064 nm/infrared	CoolGlide Vantage/ Cutera	F
Nd:YAG &	1064 nm/infrared	CoolGlide XEO/Cutera	F
Intense Pulsed Light	& 600-850 nm/IPL		B
Nd:YAG	1064 nm/infrared	Lyra/Laserscope	F
Nd:YAG	1064 nm/infrared	Varia/CoolTouch	F
Nd:YAG	1064 nm/infrared	Profile/Sciton	F
Nd:YAG	1064 nm/infrared	VascuLight Elite/ Lumenis	F
Intense Pulsed Light	1064 nm/infrared	IPL Quantum DL/ Lumenis	F
Nd:YAG	1064 nm/infrared	GentleYAG/Candela	F
Q-switched Nd:YAG	1064 nm/infrared	MedLite C6/HOYA	B
	& 532 nm/green		A
Q-switched Nd:YAG	1064 nm/infrared	MedLite C3/HOYA	B
	& 532 nm/green		A

Q-switched Nd:YAG	532 nm/green	Q-YAG 5/Palomar	A
	& 1064 nm/infrared		B
Nd:YAG	1320 nm/infrared	CoolTouch/CoolTouch	F
Diode	800 nm	LightSheer/Lumenis	F
Carbon dioxide (CO2)	10,600 nm/infrared	Encore/Lumenis	A-
CO2	10,600 nm/infrared	Ultrapulse/Lumenis	A-
Erbium:YAG	2940 nm/infrared	Venus/Laserscope	A-
Erbium:YAG	2940 nm/infrared	Profile Contour/Sciton	A-
Erbium:YAG	2940 nm/infrared	Burane SL/WaveLight	A-
Erbium:YAG	2940 nm/infrared	Harmony/Orion (Alma)	A-
Erbium:YAG	2940 nm/infrared	Whisper/Radiancy	A-
Fiber laser	1550 nm/infrared	Fraxel SR/Reliant	B

Performing excellent facial skin rejuvenation is an art and science. This is the one procedure that completely separates the amateurs from the pros. A top-trained doctor will know how to treat the eye area and over the eyelids safely without causing harm to the eyes. Amateurs will hopefully avoid the eye area because they realize their limitations. The dangerous amateurs will not recognize their own ignorance and may attempt to treat the eye area and cause serious damage. Some lasers are safe to use around the eye area with appropriate eye protection and others are completely contraindicated over the eye area.

I remember when the salesmen for CoolTouch and NLite lasers were telling physicians that they could safely treat over the eyelids without any eye protection. I knew that this was not accurate but many doctors did not and just assumed the laser reps knew what they were talking about. I also remember when the IPL salesmen were telling everyone they didn't need to use eye protection on themselves (the operator) or the patients. Many physicians and nurses have absolutely no training in this area at all and are misinformed by the laser company and become quite cavalier. The problem is they're so ignorant that they don't even realize how much they don't know. These are the most dangerous people of all.

The big problem with the laser industry is that sometimes the laser company themselves are not aware of some safety hazards and do not have the proper medical background to be able to make sound clinical judgments. They are not physicians. However, they peddle their medical devices to physicians who are not trained or skilled in this particular field so it is like the blind leading the blind. It is a problem evolving from pure economics. If laser companies only sold to qualified physicians, they wouldn't be in business for very long. Doctors formally trained in lasers are a rare breed and could not provide enough business to sustain the laser industry. As a result, laser companies have sold the vast majority of their devices to completely unqualified and untrained professionals. Most of these individuals start performing laser treatments after only attending a weekend seminar.

I have seen patients who told me that their other doctor who treated them had told them it wasn't possible to treat the eye area. I told them they were lucky that the physician didn't attempt to since they were obviously not trained to do this. But it was improper for that doctor to tell them that it was "impossible" to treat the eye area (they just didn't want to refer them to a qualified laser surgeon who would know how to treat the eye area).

The ratings for skin photorejuvenation are based upon the laser's ability to remove both vascular and pigmented lesions. Another factor taken into consideration for the rating is the laser's effect on collagen stimulation that helps the facial skin look firmer and feel smoother to the touch (tone and texture). Wrinkle reduction is a bonus but not a major criteria in this category. Many lasers touted the ability to remove wrinkles as well as sun damage. In reality, the amount of wrinkle reduction resulting from noninvasive laser rejuvenation has been disappointing — even more disappointing with light and LED devices. So I have created a separate comparison chart to look just at wrinkle reduction. (See comparison chart for "Wrinkle Reduction"). The major factor in rating the photorejuvenation category was assessing the laser's effectiveness and safety in terms of treating the entire face and other body parts. Laser systems that have more than one laser contained within its console received a rating based on the use of all lasers contained within that console.

Also, some systems, which were rated very high for treating individual pigmented lesions, may receive lower ratings for skin photorejuvenation because they don't possess adequate cooling in order to safely treat over the entire face on all skin types.

Top Lasers for Noninvasive Photorejuvenation:

1. 532 nm/KTP (green) laser
   Brand/Company: Gemini/Laserscope (A+), Aura/Laserscope (A), Versapulse/Lumenis (A), Diolite/Iridex (A-)

2. Intense Pulsed Light + Bipolar radiofrequency
   Aurora/Syneron (B)

3. Intense Pulsed Light
   560LP/Cutera (B), EsteLux/Palomar (B-), Quantum/Lumenis (B-)

4. 585 nm/Pulsed dye (yellow) laser
   Vbeam/Candela (C+)

Comparison Chart for Noninvasive Skin Photorejuvenation

Class or Type of Laser	Wavelength/Color	Brand Name/Company	Grade
Pulsed dye laser	595 nm/yellow	Vbeam/Candela	C+
Pulsed dye laser	585 nm/yellow	Cbeam/Candela	C+
Pulsed dye laser	585 nm/yellow	Photogenica/Cynosure	C+
Pulsed dye laser	585-595 nm/yellow	Sclerolase/Candela	C+
Pulsed dye laser	585 nm/yellow	NLite/ICN	D
Intense Pulse Light &	500-950 nm/IPL	Cynergy 3/Cynosure	B-
Nd:YAG &	& 1064 nm/infrared		D
Pulsed dye laser	& 595 nm/yellow		C+
KTP and	532 nm/green &	Gemini/Laserscope	A+
Nd:YAG	1064 nm/infrared		D
KTP	532 nm/green	Aura/Laserscope	A
KTP	532 nm/green	Diolite/Iridex	A-
KTP and	532 nm/green &	VariLite/Iridex	A
Diode	940 nm/infrared		D
KTP	532 nm/green	Versapulse/Lumenis	A

Intense Pulsed Light	400-1400 nm/IPL	StarLux/Palomar	B-
and Nd:YAG laser	& 1064 nm/infrared		D
Intense Pulsed Light	400-1400 nm/IPL	MediLux/Palomar	B-
Intense Pulsed Light	400-1400 nm/IPL	EsteLux/Palomar	B-
Intense Pulsed Light	560-1200 nm/IPL	IPL Quantum SR/ Lumenis	B-
Intense Pulsed Light	515-1200 nm/IPL	VascuLight Elite/ Lumenis	B-
Intense Pulsed Light	515-1200 nm/IPL	Lumenis One/Lumenis	B-
Intense Pulsed Light	600-850 nm/IPL	CoolGlide XEO/Cutera	B-
Intense Pulsed Light	560 nm/IPL	560LP/Cutera	B
Intense Pulsed Light	500-610 nm/IPL	Clareon VR/Novalis	B-
Intense Pulsed Light	520-1200 nm/IPL	Solarus VR/Novalis	B-
Pulsed Light + Radiofrequency	580-980 nm/IPL	Aurora SR/Syneron	B
Diode + Radiofrequency	900 nm	Polaris Vascular/Syneron	D
Light Heat Energy	400-1200 nm/IPL	SkinStation/Radiancy	B-
Nd:YAG	1064 nm/infrared	CoolGlide Excel/Cutera	D
Nd:YAG	1064 nm/infrared	CoolGlide Vantage/ Cutera	D
Nd:YAG & Intense Pulsed Light	1064 nm/infrared & 600-850 nm/IPL	CoolGlide XEO/Cutera	D B-
Nd:YAG	1064 nm/infrared	Lyra/Laserscope	D
Nd:YAG	1064 nm/infrared	Varia/CoolTouch	D
Nd:YAG	1064 nm/infrared	Profile/Sciton	D
Nd:YAG	1064 nm/infrared	VascuLight Elite/ Lumenis	D
Intense Pulsed Light & Nd:YAG	560-1200 nm/IPL +1064 nm/infrared	IPL Quantum DL/ Lumenis	B- D
Nd:YAG	1064 nm/infrared	GentleYAG/Candela	D
Q-switched Nd:YAG	1064 nm/infrared & 532 nm/green	MedLite C6/HOYA	C- C+
Q-switched Nd:YAG	1064 nm/infrared & 532 nm/green	MedLite C3/HOYA	C- C+
Q-switched Nd:YAG	532 nm/green & 1064 nm/infrared	Q-YAG 5/Palomar	C+ C-

| Nd:YAG | 1320 nm/infrared | CoolTouch/CoolTouch | D |
| Fiber laser | 1550 nm/infrared | Fraxel SR/Reliant | C+ |

WRINKLE REDUCTION

There was an incredible amount of hype associated with some non-invasive lasers that were touted as being the "holy grail" for removing wrinkles. These lasers were nonablative or noninvasive (causing no injury to the skin) and were supposed to remove wrinkles to the same extent as the invasive CO2 laser. The CO2 laser is the gold standard for smoothing wrinkles but it has the major disadvantage of having a long recovery time and increased side effects and complications, especially if performed by an untrained physician. The CO2 tidal wave took the nation by storm in the early 90's—people were getting their faces resurfaced in massive numbers. Everyone thought they had found the fountain of youth. But then there were lots of complications and patients complained of looking red and sunburned too long—so they clamored for something noninvasive. Along came the NLite and CoolTouch in 1999 and 2000—these were the first noninvasive lasers that claimed to produce CO2 results without any downtime at all.

Many dermatologists, including well-known leaders in the field, got caught up with the hype. They got on the gravy train to be paid consultants and speakers for the laser companies to promote these devices to other physicians. In time, we all learned that the results were far less than the hype. In fact, it was a case of the emperor's new clothes and physicians began to wonder, when will everyone else realize that the emperor has no clothes on? Not only were the NLite and CoolTouch not the Holy Grail, but also it became questionable whether these lasers produced any results at all.

Now the same thing is occurring with the Fraxel laser. It has been hyped again as the "holy grail"—a laser that produces CO2 results without any downtime. Once again, that has not panned out. The word Holy Grail has been so overused in the cosmetic laser field that it no longer carries any real meaning. I cringe when anyone even uses this term because it immediately arouses skepticism within me. The Fraxel laser is an improvement over the NLite and CoolTouch lasers but inferior to the CO_2 and Erbium lasers. It doesn't produce CO_2 results and it does have some downtime. It's not really noninvasive nor is it truly invasive—it lies in a nebulous region in-between. The results are also somewhere in-between. When it comes to wrinkle reduction, the more injury there is to the skin, the better the results. There is no way to remove a wrinkle without causing injury to the skin. That's why it makes sense when the Fraxel people say that you can improve upon the results if you turn up the settings in order to injure the skin more like the CO_2 or Erbium lasers—but that raises the question as to why you should even bother with the Fraxel when you can get better results with CO_2 or Erbium laser with the same amount of downtime. The presumed reason to use the Fraxel was to deliver CO_2 results without any downtime. If you have to turn up the settings to get better results but get more downtime, why not just stick with the CO_2 laser? The Fraxel is used for fractional resurfacing which also results in a fraction of the results.

For wrinkles, the effectiveness of lasers are as follows:

CO_2 > Erbium:YAG > PSR[3] > Fraxel > NLite or CoolTouch or other nonablative lasers

Their effectiveness also corresponds to degree of injury:

CO_2 > Erbium:YAG > PSR[3] > Fraxel > NLite or CoolTouch or other nonablative lasers

The CO_2 and Erbium lasers can also be turned down to lower settings to produce less downtime and therefore less results. The Fraxel laser also has the limitation of not being able to treat over the eyelids and that's where most people want to have treatment. The CO_2 and Erbium lasers can be used to treat over the eyelids but not the Fraxel.

Top Lasers for Wrinkle Reduction

1. Carbon dioxide (CO2) laser
   Brand name/Company: Encore/Lumenis (A+), Ultrapulse/Lumenis (A+)

2. Erbium:YAG laser
   Venus/Laserscope (B+), Profile/Sciton (B+)

Comparison Chart for Wrinkle Reduction

Class or Type of Laser	Wavelength/Color	Brand Name/Company	Grade
Pulsed dye laser	595 nm/yellow	Vbeam/Candela	D+
Pulsed dye laser	585 nm/yellow	Cbeam/Candela	D+
Pulsed dye laser	585 nm/yellow	Photogenica/Cynosure	D+
Pulsed dye laser	585-595 nm/yellow	Sclerolase/Candela	D+
Pulsed dye laser	585 nm/yellow	NLite/ICN	D+
Diode	1450 nm/infrared	Smoothbeam/Candela	D+
Intense Pulse Light &	500-950 nm/IPL	Cynergy 3/Cynosure	D-
Nd:YAG &	& 1064 nm/infrared		D+
Pulsed dye laser	& 595 nm/yellow		D+
KTP and	532 nm/green &	Gemini/Laserscope	D+
Nd:YAG	1064 nm/infrared		D+
KTP	532 nm/green	Aura/Laserscope	D+
KTP	532 nm/green	Diolite/Iridex	D
KTP and	532 nm/green &	VariLite/Iridex	D
Diode	940 nm/infrared		D
KTP	532 nm/green	Versapulse/Lumenis	D+
Intense Pulsed Light	400-1400 nm/IPL	StarLux/Palomar	D-
and Nd:YAG laser	& 1064 nm/infrared		D+
Intense Pulsed Light	400-1400 nm/IPL	MediLux/Palomar	D-
Intense Pulsed Light	400-1400 nm/IPL	EsteLux/Palomar	D-
Intense Pulsed Light	560-1200 nm/IPL	IPL Quantum SR/ Lumenis	D-
Intense Pulsed Light	515-1200 nm/IPL	VascuLight Elite/Lumenis	D-
Intense Pulsed Light	515-1200 nm/IPL	Lumenis One/Lumenis	D-

Intense Pulsed Light	600-850 nm/IPL	CoolGlide XEO/Cutera	D-
Intense Pulsed Light	560 nm/IPL	560LP/Cutera	D-
Intense Pulsed Light	500-610 nm/IPL	Clareon VR/Novalis	D-
Intense Pulsed Light	520-1200 nm/IPL	Solarus VR/Novalis	D-
Pulsed Light + Radiofrequency	580-980 nm/IPL	Aurora SR/Syneron	D+
Diode + Radiofrequency	900 nm	Polaris Vascular/Syneron	C-
Light Heat Energy	400-1200 nm/IPL	SkinStation/Radiancy	D-
Nd:YAG	1064 nm/infrared	CoolGlide Excel/Cutera	D+
Nd:YAG	1064 nm/infrared	CoolGlide Vantage/Cutera	D+
Nd:YAG & Intense Pulsed Light	1064 nm/infrared & 600-850 nm/IPL	CoolGlide XEO/Cutera	D+ D-
Nd:YAG	1064 nm/infrared	Lyra/Laserscope	D+
Nd:YAG	1064 nm/infrared	Varia/CoolTouch	D+
Nd:YAG	1064 nm/infrared	Profile/Sciton	D+
Nd:YAG	1064 nm/infrared	VascuLight Elite/Lumenis	D+
Intense Pulsed Light + Nd:YAG	560-1200 nm/IPL + 1064 nm/infrared	IPL Quantum DL/ Lumenis	D- D-
Nd:YAG	1064 nm/infrared	GentleYAG/Candela	D+
Q-switched Nd:YAG	1064 nm/infrared & 532 nm/green	MedLite C6/HOYA	D D
Q-switched Nd:YAG	1064 nm/infrared & 532 nm/green	MedLite C3/HOYA	D D
Q-switched Nd:YAG	532 nm/green & 1064 nm/infrared	Q-YAG 5/Palomar	D D
Nd:YAG	1320 nm/infrared	CoolTouch/CoolTouch	D+
Diode	800 nm	LightSheer/Lumenis	D
Carbon dioxide (CO2)	10,600 nm/infrared	Encore/Lumenis	A+
CO2	10,600 nm/infrared	Ultrapulse/Lumenis	A+
Erbium:YAG	2940 nm/infrared	Venus/Laserscope	B+
Erbium:YAG	2940 nm/infrared	Profile Contour/Sciton	B+
Erbium:YAG	2940 nm/infrared	Burane SL/WaveLight	B
Erbium:YAG	2940 nm/infrared	Harmony/Orion (Alma)	B
Erbium:YAG	2940 nm/infrared	Whisper/Radiancy	B
Plasma + Radiofrequency	Nitrogen plasma	PSR³/Rhytec/Gyrus	B-

| Fiber laser | 1550 nm/infrared | Fraxel SR/Reliant | C |
| Radiofrequency | | ThermaCool/Thermage | C- |

Top Lasers for Skin Tightening:

1. Monopolar Radiofrequency
   Brand/Company: ThermaCool/Thermage (A-)

2. Infrared Light
   Titan/Cutera (B)

Comparison Chart for Skin Tightening

Class or Type of Laser	Wavelength/Color	Brand Name/Company	Grade
Pulsed dye laser	595 nm/yellow	Vbeam/Candela	C-
Pulsed dye laser	585 nm/yellow	Cbeam/Candela	C-
Pulsed dye laser	585 nm/yellow	Photogenica/Cynosure	C-
Pulsed dye laser	585-595 nm/yellow	Sclerolase/Candela	C-
Pulsed dye laser	585 nm/yellow	NLite/ICN	C-
Diode	1450 nm/infrared	Smoothbeam/Candela	C-
Intense Pulse Light &	500-950 nm/IPL	Cynergy 3/Cynosure	D-
Nd:YAG &	& 1064 nm/infrared		D
Pulsed dye laser	& 595 nm/yellow		D
KTP and	532 nm/green &	Gemini/Laserscope	C-
Nd:YAG	1064 nm/infrared		C-
KTP	532 nm/green	Aura/Laserscope	C-
KTP	532 nm/green	Diolite/Iridex	D+
KTP and	532 nm/green &	VariLite/Iridex	D+
Diode	940 nm/infrared		D+
KTP	532 nm/green	Versapulse/Lumenis	C-
Intense Pulsed Light	400-1400 nm/IPL	StarLux/Palomar	D-
and Nd:YAG laser	& 1064 nm/ infrared		C-
Intense Pulsed Light	400-1400 nm/IPL	MediLux/Palomar	D-
Intense Pulsed Light	400-1400 nm/IPL	EsteLux/Palomar	D-

Intense Pulsed Light	560-1200 nm/IPL	IPL Quantum SR/ Lumenis	D-
Intense Pulsed Light	515-1200 nm/IPL	VascuLight Elite/Lumenis	D-
Intense Pulsed Light	515-1200 nm/IPL	Lumenis One/Lumenis	D-
Intense Pulsed Light	600-850 nm/IPL	CoolGlide XEO/Cutera	D-
Intense Pulsed Light	560 nm/IPL	560LP/Cutera	D-
Intense Pulsed Light	500-610 nm/IPL	Clareon VR/Novalis	D-
Intense Pulsed Light	520-1200 nm/IPL	Solarus VR/Novalis	D-
Pulsed Light + Radiofrequency	580-980 nm/IPL	Aurora SR/Syneron	C-
Diode + Radiofrequency	900 nm	Polaris Vascular/Syneron	C+
Light Heat Energy	400-1200 nm/IPL	SkinStation/Radiancy	D-
Nd:YAG	1064 nm/infrared	CoolGlide Excel/Cutera	C-
Nd:YAG	1064 nm/infrared	CoolGlide Vantage/ Cutera	C-
Nd:YAG & Intense Pulsed Light	1064 nm/infrared & 600-850 nm/ IPL	CoolGlide XEO/Cutera	C- D-
Nd:YAG	1064 nm/infrared	Lyra/Laserscope	C-
Nd:YAG	1064 nm/infrared	Varia/CoolTouch	C-
Nd:YAG	1064 nm/infrared	Profile/Sciton	C-
Nd:YAG	1064 nm/infrared	VascuLight Elite/Lumenis	C-
Intense Pulsed Light & Nd:YAG	560-1200 nm/IPL &1064 nm/infrared	IPL Quantum DL/ Lumenis	D- C-
Nd:YAG	1064 nm/infrared	GentleYAG/Candela	C-
Q-switched Nd:YAG	1064 nm/infrared & 532 nm/green	MedLite C6/HOYA	D D
Q-switched Nd:YAG	1064 nm/infrared & 532 nm/green	MedLite C3/HOYA	D D
Q-switched Nd:YAG	532 nm/green & 1064 nm/ infrared	Q-YAG 5/Palomar	D D
Nd:YAG	1320 nm/infrared	CoolTouch/CoolTouch	C-
Diode	800 nm	LightSheer/Lumenis	C-
Carbon dioxide (CO2)	10,600 nm/infrared	Encore/Lumenis	B+
CO2	10,600 nm/infrared	Ultrapulse/Lumenis	B+

Erbium:YAG	2940 nm/infrared	Venus/Laserscope	B-
Erbium:YAG	2940 nm/infrared	Profile Contour/Sciton	B-
Erbium:YAG	2940 nm/infrared	Burane SL/WaveLight	B-
Erbium:YAG	2940 nm/infrared	Harmony/Orion (Alma)	B-
Erbium:YAG	2940 nm/infrared	Whisper/Radiancy	B-
Fiber laser	1550 nm/infrared	Fraxel SR/Reliant	C
Radiofrequency		ThermaCool/Thermage	A-
Pulsed Light	1100-1800 nm/ infrared	Titan/Cutera	B

TOP LASERS FOR ACNE:

1. 532 nm/KTP (green) laser
   Brand/Company: Gemini/Laserscope (A+), Aura/Laserscope (A), Versapulse/ Lumenis (A)

2. 1450 nm/Diode (infrared) laser
   Smoothbeam/Candela (A)

3. Monopolar Radiofrequency
   ThermaCool/Thermage (A)

4. 585 or 595 nm/Pulsed dye (yellow) laser
   Vbeam/Candela (A-), NLite/ICN (A-)

5. 1064 nm/Nd:YAG (infrared) laser
   Lyra/Laserscope (A-), Varia/CoolTouch (A-), CoolGlide/ Cutera (B+)

6. 900 nm/Diode + Bipolar Radiofrequency
   Polaris/Syneron (A-)

7. Blue Light + Intense Pulsed Light + Bipolar Radiofrequency
   Galaxy/Syneron (B)

8. Intense Pulsed Light + Bipolar Radiofrequency
   Aurora/Syneron (B-)

COMPARISON CHART FOR ACNE

Class or Type of Laser	Wavelength/Color	Brand Name/Company	Grade
Pulsed dye laser	595 nm/yellow	Vbeam/Candela	A-
Pulsed dye laser	585 nm/yellow	Cbeam/Candela	B+
Pulsed dye laser	585 nm/yellow	Photogenica/Cynosure	A-
Pulsed dye laser	585-595 nm/yellow	Sclerolase/Candela	A-
Pulsed dye laser	585 nm/yellow	NLite/ICN	A-
Diode	1450 nm/infrared	Smoothbeam/Candela	A
Intense Blue Light	405-420 nm/blue	Clear 100/Lumenis	C-
Intense Blue Light	417 nm/blue	ClearLight/Lumenis	C-
Blue & White Light	400-1200 nm/IPL	Omnilight FPL/Amer Med Bio Care	C-
Blue & White Light	400-1200 nm/IPL	Novalight FPL/Amer Med Bio Care	C-
LED	417 nm/blue	OmniLux/Cutera	C-
Blue Light	417 nm/blue	BLU-U/DUSA	C-
*5-ALA (Levulan) and BLU-U	417 nm/blue	BLU-U/DUSA	B
Intense Pulse Light & Nd:YAG & Pulsed dye laser	500-950 nm/IPL & 1064 nm/infrared & 595 nm/yellow	Cynergy 3/Cynosure	C- A- A-
KTP and Nd:YAG	532 nm/green & 1064 nm/infrared	Gemini/Laserscope	A+ A-
KTP	532 nm/green	Aura/Laserscope	A
KTP	532 nm/green	Diolite/Iridex	A-
KTP and Diode	532 nm/green & 940 nm/infrared	VariLite/Iridex	A- A-
KTP	532 nm/green	Versapulse/Lumenis	A
Intense Pulsed Light and Nd:YAG laser	400-1400 nm/IPL & 1064 nm/infrared	StarLux/Palomar	C- A-
Intense Pulsed Light	400-1400 nm/IPL	MediLux/Palomar	C-
Intense Pulsed Light	400-1400 nm/IPL	EsteLux/Palomar	C-
Intense Pulsed Light	560-1200 nm/IPL	IPL Quantum SR/Lumenis	C-
Intense Pulsed Light	515-1200 nm/IPL	VascuLight Elite/Lumenis	C-

Intense Pulsed Light	515-1200 nm/IPL	Lumenis One/Lumenis	C-
Intense Pulsed Light	600-850 nm/IPL	CoolGlide XEO/Cutera	C-
Intense Pulsed Light	560 nm/IPL	560LP/Cutera	C-
Intense Pulsed Light	500-610 nm/IPL	Clareon VR/Novalis	C-
Intense Pulsed Light	520-1200 nm/IPL	Solarus VR/Novalis	C-
Intense Pulsed Light & Radiofrequency	580-980 nm/IPL	Aurora SR/Syneron	B-
Blue Light & IPL & Radiofrequency	400-980 nm/IPL	Galaxy/Syneron	B
Diode + Radiofrequency	900 nm/infrared	Polaris Vascular/Syneron	A-
Light Heat Energy	400-1200 nm/IPL	SkinStation/Radiancy	C-
Nd:YAG	1064 nm/infrared	CoolGlide Excel/Cutera	B+
Nd:YAG	1064 nm/infrared	CoolGlide Vantage/Cutera	B+
Nd:YAG & Intense Pulsed Light	1064 nm/infrared & 600-850 nm/IPL	CoolGlide XEO/Cutera	B+ C-
Nd:YAG	1064 nm/infrared	Lyra/Laserscope	A-
Nd:YAG	1064 nm/infrared	Varia/CoolTouch	A-
Nd:YAG	1064 nm/infrared	Profile/Sciton	B+
Nd:YAG	1064 nm/infrared	VascuLight Elite/Lumenis	A-
Intense Pulsed Light & Nd:YAG	560-1200 nm/IPL & 1064 nm/infrared	IPL Quantum DL/ Lumenis	C- A-
Nd:YAG	1064 nm/infrared	GentleYAG/Candela	A-
Nd:YAG	1320 nm/infrared	CoolTouch/CoolTouch	A-
Diode	800 nm	LightSheer/Lumenis	A-
Radiofrequency		ThermaCool/Thermage	A

5-Aminolevulinic Acid (5-ALA), also known as Levulan (DUSA), is a chemical that is applied to the acne lesions and then activated by a light source to active the chemical. Using 5-ALA with any laser or light or LED source helps get better acne clearance faster. The problem with using 5-ALA is that it causes increased sun sensitivity so the patient will have several days of redness and need to stay out of the sun. This is difficult for many teenagers who are active in sports. The reason many teenagers look for options to being on oral antibiotics and isotretinoin (Accutane) is to avoid increased sun sensitivity and other side effects. Lasers are more effective than light or

LED at treating acne because the laser beam penetrates deeper to the oil glands to shrink the oil glands and to kill the bacteria. Using an effective laser may not require usage of 5-ALA. Since light and LED devices don't penetrate deep enough in the skin to be as effective against acne, 5-ALA becomes a more necessary adjunct if one desires better acne clearance.

Light and LED treatments are less costly than laser treatments. Light treatments generally cost about $150 a treatment. Laser treatments can cost $350 to $750 a treatment on average. Adding 5-ALA would add an additional cost of $100 to $150 to the treatment.

Top Lasers for Hair Removal
(White skin, dark hair):

1. 770-1100 nm/Intense Pulsed Light
   ProWave770/Cutera (A+)

2. 755 nm/Alexandrite (near infrared) laser
   GentleLASE/Candela (A+)

3. 800 nm/Diode (infrared) laser
   LightSheer/Lumenis (A)

4. Intense Pulsed Light + Bipolar Radiofrequency
   Aurora/Syneron (A)

Comparison Chart for Hair Removal
(White skin, dark hair)

Class or Type of Laser	Wavelength/Color	Brand Name/Company	Grade
Alexandrite	755 nm/infrared	GentleLASE/Candela	A+
Alexandrite	755 nm/infrared	Apogee/Cynosure	A-
Diode	800 nm/infrared	LightSheer/Lumenis	A
Intense Pulsed Light	770-1100 nm/IPL	ProWave770/Cutera	A+
Diode + vacuum	810 nm/infrared	PPX/Aesthera	C
KTP and Nd:YAG	532 nm/green & 1064 nm/infrared	Gemini/Laserscope	B-

KTP and Diode	532 nm/green & 940 nm/infrared	VariLite/Iridex	B-
Diode	800 nm	Apex 800/Iridex	A-
Intense Pulsed Light	400-1400 nm/IPL	StarLux/Palomar	B
Intense Pulsed Light	400-1400 nm/IPL	MediLux/Palomar	B
Intense Pulsed Light	400-1400 nm/IPL	EsteLux/Palomar	B
Intense Pulsed Light	560-1200 nm/IPL	IPL Quantum SR/ Lumenis	B
Intense Pulsed Light	515-1200 nm/IPL	VascuLight Elite/Lumenis	B
Intense Pulsed Light	515-1200 nm/IPL	Lumenis One/Lumenis	B
Intense Pulsed Light	600-850 nm/IPL	CoolGlide XEO/Cutera	B
Intense Pulsed Light	630-1200 nm/IPL	Clareon/Novalis	B
Intense Pulsed Light	630-1200 nm/IPL	Solarus VR/Novalis	B
Intense Pulsed Light		Solis/Laserscope	B
Pulsed Light + Radiofrequency	680-980 nm/IPL	Aurora DSR/Syneron	A
Diode + Radiofrequency	810 nm	Polaris DS Comet/Syneron	A
Pulsed Light + Diode + Radiofrequency	580-980 nm/IPL & 810 nm/infrared	Galaxy/Syneron	A
Light Heat Energy	400-1200 nm/IPL	SkinStation/Radiancy	B
Nd:YAG	1064 nm/infrared	CoolGlide Excel/Cutera	B
Nd:YAG	1064 nm/infrared	CoolGlide Vantage/Cutera	B
Nd:YAG & IPL	1064 nm/infrared & 600-850 nm/IPL	CoolGlide XEO/Cutera	B
Nd:YAG	1064 nm/infrared	Lyra/Laserscope	B-
Nd:YAG	1064 nm/infrared	Varia/Lumenis	B-
Nd:YAG	1064 nm/infrared	Profile/Sciton	B-
Nd:YAG	1064 nm/infrared	Lumenis One/Lumenis	B-
Intense Pulsed Light	515-1200 nm/IPL	Lumenis One/Lumenis	B
LightSheer Diode	800 nm/infrared	Lumenis One/Lumenis	A-
Nd:YAG	1064 nm/infrared	GentleYAG/Candela	B-

Top Lasers for Hair Removal (Dark skin, dark hair):

1. Long-pulsed 1064 nm/Nd:YAG (infrared) laser
    Brand/Company: Lyra/Laserscope (A+), Gemini/Laserscope
    (A+), CoolGlide/Cutera (A-), Varia/CoolTouch (A-), Profile/
    Sciton (A-), GentleYAG/Candela (A-)

Comparison Chart for Hair Removal
(Dark skin, dark hair)

Class or Type of Laser	Wavelength/Color	Brand Name/Company	Grade
Alexandrite	755 nm/infrared	GentleLASE/Candela	C-
Alexandrite	755 nm/infrared	Apogee/Cynosure	D+
Diode	800 nm/infrared	LightSheer/Lumenis	C-
Intense Pulsed Light	770-1100 nm/ infrared	ProWave770/Cutera	B+
KTP and Nd:YAG	532 nm/green & 1064 nm/infrared	Gemini/Laserscope	A+
KTP and Diode	532 nm/green & 940 nm/infrared	VariLite/Iridex	C+
Diode	800 nm	Apex 800/Iridex	C+
Intense Pulsed Light	400-1400 nm/IPL	StarLux/Palomar	D-
Intense Pulsed Light	400-1400 nm/IPL	MediLux/Palomar	D-
Intense Pulsed Light	400-1400 nm/IPL	EsteLux/Palomar	D-
Intense Pulsed Light	560-1200 nm/IPL	IPL Quantum SR/ Lumenis	D-
Intense Pulsed Light & Nd:YAG & Diode	515-1200 nm/IPL 1064 nm & 800 nm	Lumenis One/Lumenis	B
Intense Pulsed Light	630-1200 nm/IPL	Clareon/Novalis	D-
Intense Pulsed Light	630-1200 nm/IPL	Solarus VR/Novalis	D-
Intense Pulsed Light		Solis/Laserscope	D-
Pulsed Light + Radiofrequency	680-980 nm/IPL	Aurora DSR/Syneron	C-
Diode + Radiofrequency	810 nm	Polaris DS Comet/ Syneron	B-

Pulsed Light + Diode + Radiofrequency	580-980 nm/IPL & 810 nm/infrared	Galaxy/Syneron	C-
Light Heat Energy	400-1200 nm/IPL	SkinStation/Radiancy	D-
Nd:YAG	1064 nm/infrared	CoolGlide Excel/Cutera	A-
Nd:YAG	1064 nm/infrared	CoolGlide Vantage/ Cutera	A-
Nd:YAG & IPL	1064 nm/infrared & 600-850 nm/IPL	CoolGlide XEO/Cutera	A-
Nd:YAG	1064 nm/infrared	Lyra/Laserscope	A+
Nd:YAG	1064 nm/infrared	Varia/CoolTouch	A-
Nd:YAG	1064 nm/infrared	Profile/Sciton	A-
Nd:YAG	1064 nm/infrared	Lumenis One/Lumenis	A-
Intense Pulsed Light	515-1200 nm/IPL	Lumenis One/Lumenis	D-
LightSheer Diode	800 nm/infrared	Lumenis One/Lumenis	C-
Nd:YAG	1064 nm/infrared	GentleYAG/Candela	A-

Light brown, blonde, gray, and white hairs are less responsive to any laser treatment. Also, fine hairs (ie: peach fuzz) may be completely unresponsive. I have successfully treated patients with these hair types but usually have to perform an inordinate number of treatments and use several different laser devices in order to achieve results. The lighter and finer the hair, the more difficult the treatment. The best hair responders are always dark coarse hairs. Brown hair is less responsive than black hair. Medium density hairs are less responsive than coarse hairs. Certain regions also typically respond much faster such as underarms and bikini regions. In comparison, backs and legs respond much slower.

Patients often compare results with friends. A frequent question asked is, "Why did my friend get complete hair clearance after only one treatment and it's taking me so much longer?" It's usually due to having different hair color and type. Most likely the friend who had immediate clearance had dark coarse hairs. The person with slower clearance most likely has finer and lighter hairs. Brown hair is less responsive than black hair. Medium density hairs are less responsive than coarse hairs.

This guide is intended to help the layperson navigate through the bewildering choices of lasers. Despite the best intentions in surfing the net and reading every publication available about lasers, you will be greatly disappointed with the results if you don't choose the right doctor. Remember, the Golden Rule is: the laser is only as good as the doctor performing the treatment. An A+ laser can give C- results if the treatment is performed by a C- doctor. Conversely, a C- laser will always give C- results even if performed by an A+ doctor. However, an A+ doctor would know to combine different lasers (even if they're individually less than A+ lasers) in order to give A+ results.

REFERENCES

[1]   Anderson RR, Parrish JA, selective photothermolysis: precise microsurgery by selective absorption of pulsed radiation. Science 1983; 220: 524-7.

CHAPTER 3:
CHOOSING THE RIGHT
DOCTOR

PATIENTS COMING IN FOR anti-aging treatments are still being treated for medical conditions (even though they're classified as "cosmetic"). For example, the treatment of sun damage requires the ability to properly diagnose and distinguish between lentigos (freckles), seborrheic keratoses (liver spots) that are benign vs. malignant skin cancers and precancerous lesions. You have to be able to diagnose the problem first—otherwise you could be mistakenly treating a melanoma. (By the way, this happens frighteningly often where unqualified physicians and nonphysicians attempt to treat a pigmented lesion with a laser that they have mistaken for a freckle or mole when it is actually a melanoma.)

Many patients with rosacea or eczema or other sensitive skin problems get mistakenly treated with procedures that will aggravate their condition. But you wouldn't know how to treat them properly if you first couldn't properly diagnose their condition.

And who are best trained to diagnose skin conditions and problems? Dermatologists.

All cosmetic procedures are medical procedures. Skin-related problems are medical conditions requiring proper diagnosis and treatment even if they're considered cosmetic. You have to be able to diagnose the problem first—how do you know if that pigmented lesion is a mole or a melanoma? How do you know if the reason your skin is always so sensitive to different products is because you have rosacea or eczema? Only a dermatologist is trained in answering these questions. Dermatologists are **THE** skin specialists. Unfortunately, not every dermatologist is familiar with or trained to use lasers.

Another doctor may be familiar with lasers but know nothing of the skin. The ideal specialist to perform laser treatments would be a physician with formal training in both dermatology <u>and</u> lasers.

However, if you couldn't find a doctor who possessed formal training in both dermatology and lasers, it's still better to see a dermatologist. In the worst case scenario if a complication occurred, the dermatologist would at least know how to deal with the complications because of their knowledge of proper wound care and healing. (One caveat: as in any field or specialty, there are good and bad doctors. Some doctors do well on written exams but are inept at practicing medicine.)

Here are some basic preliminary questions to ask when selecting the proper laser practice: (1) Is the practice owned by an M.D.? (2) Is the M.D. on site at all times or does the M.D. only come in once a week or once a month? (3) Who does the treatments? (4) Where did the M.D. get their training? What is their area of specialty and most importantly, are they board-certified and what area did they receive their board-certification in? A physician may advertise that they do "cosmetic surgery" or "dermatology and skin care" but they may actually have received their training and board certification in Internal Medicine or Family Practice or Ob/Gyn. Make sure you ask them this very directly, "What did you receive your board certification in?" Do not let them sidetrack this question with vague references such as, "I specialize in lasers and cosmetics," or "I've been doing this for years," or "I've been in practice for over 30 years (yeah, right, doing OB/Gyn that is. They may have just bought their laser last month. Also, another hint, lasers are a relatively young industry—most lasers haven't even been around for 30 years). Even if they say they got their training at Stanford, probe further and find out exactly what did they train in at Stanford. They may have gone to medical school at Stanford or finished residency training in colorectal surgery, but have absolutely no formal training in lasers or cosmetic surgery or dermatology. Ask them specifically, "Where did you get your training in lasers?" Most doctors got their laser training from attending a weekend course. Very few doctors actually have formal training in lasers and cosmetic surgery.

The three most important criteria for choosing a doctor are training, skill, and experience – and none of these can be bought from a laser company.

It may shock you to discover that a doctor can claim to practice any specialty. There are no laws preventing a family practitioner from running ads claiming to perform neurosurgery, for example. They cannot claim to be a "board-certified neurosurgeon" unless they really are. But they can hang a shingle and run ads stating, "Dr. Ima Quack, specializing in neurosurgery and plastic surgery." Dr. Quack may actually be board-certified in internal medicine. And there are no laws preventing him from advertising in this manner.

If you don't remember anything else, remember this one GOLDEN RULE: If a doctor does not specifically state they are board-certified in a particular specialty, then you can assume they are not. Think about it. If you had spent many years pursuing and completing proper education and training in a given specialty, wouldn't you be proud of this and what to proclaim this to the world? You're darn right—you'd be bragging about it to everyone! You wouldn't be keeping it a secret.

Doctors like myself who have legitimate training make it obvious to our patients. The first thing that patients receive when they walk into my practice is a copy of my credentials that clearly states that I'm a board-certified dermatologist with advanced fellowship training in Mohs micrographic surgery/skin cancer surgery/reconstructive surgery, dermatologic surgery, and laser and cosmetic surgery.

If you read an ad that says, "Dr. Anybody, specializing in dermatology and plastic surgery" and there is no specific reference to being "board-certified in dermatology" or "board-certified in plastic surgery" then you can assume that they are not. Any board-certified dermatologist would place this designation very prominently on their door, any advertisements or marketing materials, their website, their brochures and written materials, the yellow pages, etc. And if this doctor is the genuine McCoy, then you will be able to find many written materials stating that this doctor is board-certified in dermatology.

If the doctor does not state they are fellowship-trained, then you can assume they are not. Any doctor who had finished their residency and went on to pursue further subspecialty training by completing a fellowship would clearly state this. A plastic surgeon who went on after his plastic surgery residency to complete a fellowship in hand surgery would proudly and prominently profess this to the world and this would be stated in all his written materials given at the office. His business card and letterhead and advertisements and informational materials would all state this clearly in writing. A fellowship-trained hand surgeon is the only specialist I'd ever allow to do major hand surgery on me.

A surgeon who went on to pursue fellowship training in cardiothoracic surgery would clearly state this in the same way. There would be no ambiguity or mystery about his or her training. Incidentally, this is the only specialist I'd ever allow to do open-heart surgery on me.

Doctors with advanced training are very proud of it and will not be shy about putting that forward. So, BEWARE of doctors who don't clearly state these things in writing. If they don't put it down in writing and make it obvious, then you can assume that they're not.

If you happened to find that a doctor was lying about his board-certification and had this documented in writing, you could forward this evidence to the state medical board and file a formal complaint against the doctor and they would take action against him.

Masqueraders can really do a number on you trying to create a façade of legitimacy. A local family practitioner in California runs ads stating that he is "board-certified" and "specializes in dermatology and cosmetic surgery". But he is very sly about not actually putting in writing that he is a "board-certified dermatologist". He can wiggle his way out of this by claiming that, "Yes, I am technically 'board-certified' (in family practice that is!), and I do 'specialize' in dermatology and cosmetic surgery." He also cites multiple organizations in which he is a member of (i.e., American Society of Cosmetic and Aesthetic Dermatology, American Society of Laser Medicine and Surgery, etc.). The name of his practice is "Advanced Dermatology, Laser and Cosmetic Surgery" (not real name). He has all sorts of official appearing certificates and plaques hanging on his wall saying he's a member of all these official sounding dermatology and laser and cosmetic surgery organizations. If you ask him what kind of doctor he is, he will reply, "I specialize in dermatology and cosmetic surgery." You will really have to work to pin him down—you'd have to specifically ask, "Are you board-certified in dermatology." If he were honest, he would have to reply, "No." If he replies, "Yes", he would be lying and the only way you could ascertain this would be if you had done your due diligence and looked him up on the American Board of Medical Specialties or California Medical Board or American Medical Association sites.

You can access these sites on-line: the American Medical Association website is: http://www.ama-assn.org/ (click on "DoctorFinder"). American Medical Association, 515 N. State St., Chicago, IL 60610. (800) 621-8335.

The California Medical Board website is: http://www.medbd. ca.gov/Lookup.htm. California Medical Board, 1426 Howe Avenue, #54, Sacramento, CA 95825. Office #: (916) 263-2382. FAX #: (916) 263-2944.

Every state has a similar state medical board in which you can request information on any doctor licensed to practice in that state.

You can find out a physician's specialty and board-certification by contacting the American Board of Medical Specialties. Their website is:

www.abms.org

(One caveat: you have to register with the site to get a password.)

There are many internists and family practitioners that are even forming professional organizations and societies with names like, "The International Society of Aesthetic and Cosmetic Dermatology" and "The Association of Anti-Aging and Cosmetic Medicine" and making themselves the President and Board of Directors of these organizations. They then issue each other citations and awards to hang on their office walls to further perpetuate the masquerade. In medicine, if doctors aren't allowed to join one organization because they're not qualified, they'll simply band together to form their own organization.

I noticed one website belonging to an internist in Los Angeles who advertises that he is the "leading expert in lasers and cosmetic surgery" and has "years of advanced training and expertise". He is the President of the "National Association of Cosmetic and Laser Surgeons" (not real name). The reason I got suspicious was that I had never heard of him. It took me 2 minutes to look him up on the AMA website and find out that he is board-certified in internal medicine and has never had any formal training in laser and cosmetic surgery.

I did further investigation about the organization that he was the President of and, lo and behold, found out that it was an organization created by him and had other internists as its members. The amazing thing is that these new "cosmetic" societies formed by internists and family practitioners are becoming bigger in numbers than the legitimate cosmetic societies. And the laser and cosmetic companies are only too eager to sponsor their conferences because it just means more revenue sources for them. Every time a new organization pops up, it's another opportunity for the laser companies to have a new market of physicians to expand into.

It doesn't matter how many professional societies and organizations a doctor claims to belong to. The only thing that matters is: what is their board-certification in? And where did they get their training?

Even the media can't always be trusted to do background checking on a doctor's background. The internist that I mentioned above who claims to be a "leading expert in lasers and cosmetic surgery" was quoted in a Los Angeles newspaper as being "the number one injector of Botox". In this article, they called him a "dermatologist" and since they didn't do any background checking which would have easily brought that falsity to light, it made me doubt whether anything else in the article was credible.

A radiologist in New York City is often quoted in magazines such as *Marie Claire* but they never mention that he is a radiologist. They call him a "cosmetic surgeon" and write about how he is an "expert in the field". He has even written a book about cosmetic surgery but no mention about being a radiologist anywhere in the book.

A well-known dermatologist who caters to celebrities and the A-list crowd in New York City does not have board-certification but this is never mentioned in any of the many magazines and TV shows that cite him as a "leading expert" in the field. He has never published any articles nor presented at any scientific meetings. He is known for giving injections of controversial substances such as silicone and Lipostabil (phosphatidylcholine) injections that purport to dissolve fat without liposuction.

Many celeb doctors appeal to them by the sheer virtue that they're willing to practice medicine at the fringes and use contraband substances that other more conservative doctors are unwilling to do so. A famous Beverly Hills doctor had a flourishing hair removal practice mostly because he was willing to write narcotic prescriptions for his celebrity clientele. He was arrested for dispensing narcotic prescriptions to a wide assortment of Hollywood celebs including Winona Ryder and Courtney Love. The celebs flocked to him because of his willingness to provide them with addictive painkillers at a price.

There are people who seek out unscrupulous doctors. They like living on the edge and don't want a straight-laced doctor who follows the rules. They test out different doctors until they find one who will do their bidding. I've gotten some strange requests from patients from that world who come in demanding completely inappropriate things and they throw a fit when I turn them down. They say things like, "Do you know who I am?" And I do, but that doesn't change the way that I practice medicine. Needless to say, I don't get on their "favorite doctor" list.

This is the same as those doctors who get on the A-list for athletes because of their willingness to give them steroids. Drug-seekers need drug dealers. Doctors who do this sort of thing are barely a step above crack pushers.

(5) If the treatment is done by a nurse or NP or PA, where did they get their training? Was it from a weekend course? Or did they get trained by their supervising M.D. And how qualified is the M.D.? (Refer to question 4). (6) How many lasers do they own? Do they just rent a laser once a month or do they own only one or 2 lasers? These are signs that they don't do very many laser treatments. And they also don't have a wide array of lasers in order to provide comprehensive services.

Practices that only have one or 2 lasers will try to push only those one or 2 lasers for everything even if they aren't the best lasers. A practice that is devoted to specializing in lasers will have a wide array of laser services and be able to customize treatments to an individual's needs instead of trying to sell everyone on a "FotoFacial."

Beware of the doctor who tries to sell you on their laser rather than their skill or training. Remember that no one laser can do it all. Also, some lasers may have some side effects, which can be easily removed by other lasers. But you would have to have access to those lasers. If you are getting laser treatments, wouldn't you want to be in the best hands with access to the widest variety of lasers so that if you did have an adverse effect from one laser, the doctor could adequately treat that side effect with other lasers? If you had a side effect with a doctor who only possesses one laser, then there's no way they can help you with certain side effects that may inevitably result no matter how careful they are.

There are ways to verify the authenticity of the information you received. If the M.D. tells you that he or she is a board-certified dermatologist, you can verify this by checking either the state medical board such as the California Medical Board or the American Medical Association or the American Board of Medical Specialties sites. On the AMA site, I looked up my own name and noticed that my name only comes up if someone uses my first and last name. If someone used my first and middle and last name (Min-Wei Christine Lee), it doesn't come up. For example, I can be pulled up by typing "M. Lee" or "Min-Wei Lee" and then it says under my name that I'm a board-certified dermatologist. If I typed in "M. Christine Lee" or "Christine Lee," my profile does not come up and I'm not listed under "Christine Lee." So it's important to get the physician's entire name and accurate spelling in order to verify information.

Do not choose doctors simply because they have impressive titles such as "Department Chair or Chief" or "President of the California Medical Association" or "Head of the Department" of an academic institution or university. Some of the worst practitioners are made chairman of the department or appointed to administrative roles. In fact, many of them are quite rusty and are no longer dedicated to solely providing patient care. Administrative roles often require time taken away from clinical responsibilities so these positions may be more attractive for a doctor who prefers administration over clinical practice. Of course, many excellent doctors are also appointed to these positions, but more often than not, the reason that doctor was appointed to the role was for reasons not related to their clinical skills.

A laser surgeon who performs thousands of laser surgeries a year is probably much more qualified than his boss who is Department Chief but "dabbles" in lasers.

There's a famous doctor who was made head of the department at the university that employed him. He's a wonderful teacher and full of knowledge and experience but I would never let him touch me with a scalpel because he doesn't perform surgery on a daily basis anymore. He was a very experienced surgeon in his heyday but has now become a "dabbler".

Doctors who perform procedures have to keep up their skills by performing these procedures on a regular and daily basis. As with any skill or profession, if you don't use it, you lose it.

Scanning through the local city newspaper, yellow pages, "Penny Saver", or other advertisements, you will find hundreds (perhaps thousands) of ads offering laser hair removal and other laser and cosmetic services. It's quite bewildering for you as a consumer to discern which are the legitimate and qualified providers. Many of the ads are for beauty and hair salons, spas, walk-in "clinics", "laser salons", and shopping malls. Some advertise having a "medical director" or physician involved, while others only list a nurse or nonphysician practitioner (R.N., N.P., P.A.). There are even more ads that don't even bother to list the names of any health practitioner.

With each passing year, I am continually astounded at the proliferation of nonphysician laser practices. They used to be the exception—they have now become the norm.

I must speak to a dozen people a day who tell me their beauty salon is now offering laser treatments along with collagen and Botox injections. One of these salons has a pediatrician who offers the clients Botox injections while they're getting their nails done and hair cut. My patients are quite prudent in turning them down. One patient said to the owner of the salon that she was not going to frequent their salon anymore because she didn't think it was proper for them to be pressuring her to do these medical procedures on her face and she told the owner, "I value my face! I would never let you touch my face with a laser!"

Many of the salon owners tell me about nurses who approach them asking them if they would like to have them come in on certain days to do laser treatments for their clients. These traveling nurses peddle their services to each salon, carting their laser around. They usually sustain themselves by having several salons contract with her for laser services. Usually the nurse was able to purchase the laser with the help of a physician, usually a retired physician who wants to get a kickback from the laser without having to do anything. The physician will help the nurse purchase the laser by providing his/her medical license number. The nurse usually pays a percentage or commission to the physician. But the doctor has no other involvement—does not help with training or supervising. In fact, usually the doctor has no knowledge of lasers at all and would be completely inept and helpless if called upon for supervision or training. The nurse usually gets her "training" by attending a weekend seminar sponsored by the laser company that sold her the laser. And that is the full extent of her training. Then she proceeds to start practicing on her friends, family, and clients.

Why has this proliferation been allowed to occur? It's understandable in states where there are no laws regulating the use of lasers, but in California there are specific laws that exist to protect the consumers from unsafe practice of medicine and laser usage. So why is it so out of control even in a state with protective laws like California?

Let's start with the safety inspectors that are supposed to be monitoring California salons. There are approximately 38,000 salons in California and only 17 safety inspectors. According to recent news reports, the safety inspectors cannot humanly do their jobs effectively. There is absolutely no way that they can even put a dent in the oversight of salons. As a result, the salons are basically free to do whatever they want. So what if they're not cleaning instruments and operating under unsanitary conditions? There's probably a higher than 98% probability that the salon you frequent has not been inspected and you would have no clue what kind of conditions they maintain. They may reuse dirty files on your nails and soak your feet in dirty basins that contain bacteria and viruses from hundreds of other clients including those with hepatitis or HIV. If you have a pedicure which involves removing the cuticles with a sharp instrument which breaks through the skin, that may be the portal to introduce a deadly infection. There have been an alarming number of reports of serious and unusual infections that have left behind permanent scars and disfigurements in many people, and resulted in hospitalizations and near death in others. Why even bother to have an agency that has the stated intention of monitoring the safety conditions within salons if they can only realistically inspect less than 10% of the existent salons? Why not eliminate the agency altogether so the consumer does not have the false perception that they are being protected. Governor Arnold Schwarzenegger has been proposing just that in California. Eliminate the agencies that aren't doing their jobs.

A myriad of horrific events occur at salons. A popular show on TV called "Nip/Tuck" had an episode in which Dr. Christian Troy (a lead character on the show who is a plastic surgeon) follows another plastic surgeon, Dr. Merrill Bobolit (who had his license revoked on a previous episode because he had been doing plastic surgery on a dog and the dog died from complications arising during surgery) into the backroom of a salon only to find that he has just killed the woman he was performing liposuction on. This episode was taken from real-life events. Fact can be stranger than fiction. I watch "Nip/Tuck" on a regular basis and feel it's more realistic than shows like "Extreme Makeover" which seems to promote only the positive aspects of cosmetic surgery.

There are numerous salons that allow liposuction to be performed in the backroom (illegally) along with other cosmetic surgical procedures. Many salons are engaged in providing medical services (also being done illegally) such as administering Botox injections, collagen and Restylane and other fillers, performing FotoFacials (also known as IPL or intense pulsed light treatments) and laser hair removal.

Many salon owners are acting as the middleman or broker to refer clients to unlicensed physicians (such as foreign doctors who are practicing medicine without a license) . They are paid a referral fee once the client signs up for a cosmetic procedure. On a recent *Dateline* segment, they had hidden cameras at a salon serving as a front for an illegal doctor from Central America who came up to recruit patients to get plastic surgery down in Costa Rica.

On a regular basis, there are reports about the FBI making arrests of illegal rings involving salons and unlicensed physicians where there have been horrible complications involved. Why not make the consumer aware that beauty salons are the Wild Wild West and anything goes? Enter at your own peril. But be prepared to suffer the consequences and if you are the victim of illegal activities (such as the illegal practice of medicine by unlicensed personnel), then you have to pay the medical costs incurred out of your own pocket. Do not make insurance companies and the American public pay for your bonehead mistakes. That should teach you to do better research before you let someone perform a procedure on you. Think twice before you go in for a pedicure. Use the legal system to sue for damages. But remove the fake facade of having a safety net because there is no safety net.

I suggest replacing the current useless agencies with a different type of enforcement agency that is completely self-funded by the penalties levied on salons and businesses that are violating clearly stated rules and regulations. First, there are laws stating that medical procedures cannot be performed in a salon (non-medical) setting. If there is a report of a violation, then an investigation is immediately carried out and if the complaint is proven to be legitimate, then a fine of $20,000 or more is levied. If the fine is not paid within 30 days, then the salon will be forced to shut down (padlocked) until it pays its fine. And each violation would be treated as such. This would create financial disincentives for salons to be engaged in the illegal practice of medicine. And then hopefully they would stick to doing hairstyling and makeup, manicures, and pedicures, which is all they should be doing anyway.

If you find yourself in a salon which is advertising doing laser hair removal or FotoFacials or offers to do Botox or collagen injections, RUN! Even if you admit that you had a momentary lapse of sanity and allowed someone at a salon to inject Botox in your forehead and did not suffer any complications, you should not be aiding and abetting that salon's ability to continue to engage in these illegal activities that will eventually harm somebody else. By financially assisting them by paying for these services, you are encouraging them to continue to render these services that they are performing illegally and will cause harm to others. It is also unfair to all the physicians and medical practices that are performing these procedures legally and legitimately who are bearing the costs of providing medical care legally by paying for licensing fees, malpractice insurance, and shouldering high overhead costs for maintaining a proper medical facility and for adhering to legal medical codes which have been instituted in order to provide for public health and safety. This is analogous to buying an occasional nickel or dime bag from a drug dealer--you may think you're just an occasional recreational drug user but you are aiding and abetting that drug dealer's ability to continue operating illegally and eventually the drugs will cause great harm to others. We will never win the war on drugs because there is an endless demand for the supply. We will never be able to stop the illegal practice of medicine within salons unless we curtail the demand. They only continue to operate because of the demand. People are constantly lured in by the convenience and cheaper prices.

I have had so many people say to me that the very reason they think lasers must be safe is because they are being done in shopping malls. They figure that if it were a medical treatment, they wouldn't be allowed to operate in malls. That's why we have laws stating that these services cannot be performed in malls—because there shouldn't be this false perception that they are simple beauty treatments—they are medical treatments which can be potentially hazardous if not performed in the proper setting. And the shopping mall is not a proper setting because of the very illusion they create of making these treatments appear nonmedical. But the problem is that these laws are not being enforced.

Another episode of "Nip/Tuck" had Dr. Merrill Bobolit doing Botox parties at the home's of rich socialites—only the Botox wasn't for the socialites but for their maids who wanted to get a chance to know what it felt to be like the rich ladies they waited on. But since they couldn't afford to see a real doctor, they welcomed the services of sleazoid doctors like Bobolit who advertised having invented his own "Bobotox" which he claimed was "better than Botox". Turns out he was injecting illegal silicone into the face of these ladies and they all showed up at Dr. Troy and McNamara's (the legitimate plastic surgeons and lead characters of the show) practice with horrible disfigurements of the face resulting from the silicone injections. Once again, this seemed to be taken directly from real-life front page headlines.

There are countless numbers of "doctors" (some licensed, many with suspended or revoked medical licenses, and many more who are foreign doctors who don't have a license to practice in the U.S., and still others who have absolutely zero medical training at all) who are eager to exploit the cosmetic field.

I applaud the creators of "Nip/Tuck" for portraying plastic and cosmetic surgery in a more realistic light, unlike "Extreme Makeover" which tries to make plastic surgery look so easy and is basically an infomercial for the plastic surgery industry. It's ironic that reality shows are not realistic at all, and that dramatized shows like "Nip/Tuck" are more "real" than any reality show ever could. The producers and writers of "Nip/Tuck" take their stories straight from the headlines—they base all their medical stories on real-life events that they cull from newspaper stories. That's why their shows have such an authentic ring.

In Hawaii, there was a ring of Korean women who advertised doing cheap plastic surgery in the newspapers—they would get a large suite at the Hyatt Regency and perform plastic surgery (breast implants and facelifts) on clients, unbeknownst to the hotel. The women had worked in various capacities (receptionist, nurses) at a plastic surgeon's office in Korea. None had ever been trained or performed surgery at the plastic surgeon's office—they had only observed these surgeries being performed. They somehow got the birdbrain idea that they could make a lot of money doing plastic surgery on the side for bargain-basement hunters. They were right in one respect: if the price is right, you'll always have potential buyers. They would do a bunch of patients and then leave town. The local ER would then start getting an influx of patients with strange complications from plastic surgery and they all gave the similar story of having had their surgery performed at the Hyatt Regency. There would be an ongoing wave of these events—each time the ring came into town, there would be a cluster of complications they would leave in their wake. Many of these patients had infections, dehiscence (splitting) of the wounds, poor wound healing, or other complications that they had no recourse to get help with because their "doctors" had left town. And the authorities were never able to press any charges because the perpetrators were foreigners and there was no way to track where they had gone.

In my local area, there were two medical assistants who worked for a plastic surgeon who snuck into his office late at night and tried performing liposuction on each other. One medical assistant (M.A.) accidentally perforated the other M.A.'s liver and she ended up in the ICU at the hospital in critical condition.

I wonder if they had successfully carried off their liposuction experiment if they might have gotten more ambitious and decided to moonlight their services to salons and other businesses to make extra cash. But that's usually how all this illegal business starts—a staff member gets it into their head that, "Hey, I think I could do that—this would be a good way for me to make money. Why should doctors be the only ones? After all, it looks so easy!"

Many nurses underestimate the complexity of decisions that occur around medical procedures. They may watch a physician perform a procedure many times and convince themselves that they could do the same thing without actually understanding all the various nuances and subtleties that go into making individual decisions. The real proof in the pudding surfaces when a complication occurs—does that person know how to handle it? Nothing in medicine ever goes 100% smoothly—there is so much individual variation in the outcome of any treatment. An experienced physician has seen every variation and complication that can occur and has learned to anticipate these and knows how to intervene. They can avoid or minimize damage by applying proper judgment. Someone who thinks something is easy is deceiving themselves based on their own ignorance. The more you know about something, the more you truly appreciate how complicated it can be.

There are just too many people who only care about the bottom-line. They care more about the bargain they're getting rather than the quality of the work. Unfortunately, this is not like buying a refrigerator, car, or any other consumer product. Unlike an actual product, the medical service is only as good as the practitioner performing the service. The laser is only as good as the doctor performing the laser treatment. An excellent laser can give mediocre results if performed by a mediocre doctor. An A+ laser can give D or F results if performed by an F doctor. A C+ laser will at best only provide C+ results even if performed by an A+ doctor because of the inherent limitations in that particular technology. Therefore, it is incumbent upon being rated an

A+ doctor that that physician understands the benefits and limitations of each particular laser. When you choose a well-qualified laser expert, you are depending upon that physician's training, knowledge, judgment and experience to be able to evaluate your skin and recommend the laser treatment that would give you the optimal results while minimizing any potential complications.

There are many who think if they can't afford going to a real doctor, they'll try to substitute a fake doctor or unqualified person to give them a cheaper treatment. But this is not like buying a fake Louis Vuitton bag—all medical treatments have a potential downside, which in some cases can be life-threatening or cause permanent mutilation and disfigurement. And unlike a fake Louis Vuitton bag, which you'll just toss aside later when you tire of it, you can't change your mind later if you're not happy with the results of the laser treatment or fake "Bobotox" that you received. Some of the most expensive mistakes occur from trying to save a few dollars. If you can't afford to have it done right, don't do it at all.

Take the case of Larry King and his wife. Lionel Ritchie's ex-wife got hooked up with a South American "doctor" who was not licensed to practice in the U.S. and was doing cosmetic injections on her celebrity friends in the bathroom of her Beverly Hills mansion. Some of her friends, including Larry King's wife, came down with complications from the injections (King's wife reportedly had lumps around her lips and difficulty talking and moving her lips) which turned out not to be collagen but silicone or some other unapproved filler substance that he used to plump up their lips. They reported the complications to the authorities and the ex-Mrs. Ritchie and her boyfriend were both arrested and charged with the illegal practice of medicine without a license.

And these are people who can afford to see the best doctors in Beverly Hills. Why would they risk their health and well-being just to save a few hundred bucks?

Many people feel an almost desperate need to be able to emulate the stars by changing their appearance with cosmetic surgery. They have the false perception that somehow if they were able to do these procedures, they too would have more glamorous lives. However, since most people can't afford to do the extreme makeovers they see on TV, they'll resort to going to the bottom-dwellers (people who prey on the less fortunate, taking advantage of their naiveté and vulnerability and lack of education). These opportunists consist of the usual suspects: down-and-out doctors (untrained, unqualified, old and retired but still trying to make a few bucks, license suspended or revoked because of incompetence, malpractice, drugs or alcohol abuse, criminal behavior, etc.), foreign doctors who don't have a license to practice in the U.S., "fake" doctors who don't have any medical training at all but are masquerading as doctors (i.e., Danny Faiello), mercenary nurses/nurse practitioners/physician assistants, beauty professionals (aestheticians, cosmetologists, beauticians, electrologists), and just-plain-normal folk looking to make a buck.

People who can't afford to do it right shouldn't do it at all. These aren't necessary procedures, for God's sake. These are **cosmetic** procedures, which by their very definition are not necessary, considered luxuries, and elective/optional. People do not **need** to have any of these procedures. They are not medically necessary. However, it is absolutely necessary for your health that if you are to elect to have one of these cosmetic procedures that you do so safely without jeopardizing your health.

I see many people who are victims of botched up cosmetic surgery performed by less than qualified personnel. At best they feel they were gypped out of their money. At worst, they have permanent disfigurements and complications that they will have as a constant reminder of their lapse of judgment. And they often take on much higher costs trying to reverse what was done to them than they would have spent if they had just had it done properly to begin with. For example, it takes thousands of dollars to try to reverse the scars caused by improperly performed laser procedures. And the money they saved by going to unqualified personnel was not that significant to begin with—it pales in comparison to how much more they have to spend later to try to reverse these complications. And that's if they're even lucky enough to have the complications reversed. Many of the complications are completely irreversible no matter how much money they would want to spend to reverse it. And do I need to mention that there is no price tag for the value of a life. And many people suffer the most irreversible complication of all just from trying to save a few hundred or thousand dollars—the loss of their own life.

There are some specific questions you should ask when choosing the right doctor. Remember that the laser is only as good as the person operating it. There are various laws governing laser usage that differ amongst the 50 states. There is no uniformity in the law between states and in some states there are little or no laws at all governing the usage of lasers. California, New York, and New Jersey are amongst the better regulated states. They have laws on the books specifying who can own and operate lasers, how laser practices need to be supervised, and laser safety guidelines. I will be speaking mostly about California and its laws.

California has some of the most comprehensive laser laws in the United States. However, there is an extreme lack of enforcement of the laws. A chapter in this book is devoted entirely to the lack of enforcement and regulation of laser practices. (See Chapter 4).

In California, only a physician may purchase or own a laser device. The physician may choose to delegate laser procedures to another health professional (registered nurse, nurse practitioner, or physician assistant) to be used under proper supervision. The definition of proper supervision is the subject of some debate. At the minimum, the physician needs to be able to be reached by electronic means (phone or pager). New Jersey is more stringent in this regard—they require that only physicians can use or operate lasers. New Jersey physicians cannot delegate lasers to other personnel.

As a responsible and ethical physician, I believe that the definition of appropriate supervision means that the physician is properly trained and qualified to operate lasers, that the physician has properly trained the health professional (R.N., N.P., P.A.) to be competent and qualified to operate the laser, and that the physician is either physically on the premises or within close proximity so that in the case of emergency, the physician can be notified immediately and reach the laser site within a short period of time.

In my practice, I have some laser procedures (not all) delegated to an R.N. and a P.A. It takes me at least 3 months to train a competent licensed health professional to have some bare rudimentary knowledge of lasers. It takes about a year for me to feel that a nurse or P.A. has reached a level of competency that they can start to have some autonomy and have become more proficient. During this whole time, I evaluate all patients with the nurse or P.A., review all cases, and supervise all treatments. After reviewing each patient, I go over the proper laser settings and parameters, the treatments are carried out according to my specifications. As time goes on and they become more familiar with each patient's individual response, then I don't need to see each patient prior to every treatment. I review over every patient's treatment and follow his or her progress along with the nurse or P.A. As time goes on, I have the nurse or P.A. suggest the treatment parameters but I still evaluate and review every patient with them, and we decide on the treatment parameters together. But nothing happens in my laser clinic that I did not expressly review and authorize. If there are any side effects, I am called into the room to examine the patient and recommend proper treatments and make adjustments to the laser settings.

The rules in California were meant to allow physicians the ability to delegate certain procedures to proper health professionals. The key is to have **proper** supervision. What I consider proper delegation and supervision is that the physician has complete understanding of all laser procedures, proper laser technique, and ability to diagnose and treat any and all side effects or complications that could occur during these procedures. Then the physician has the responsibility of ensuring quality control if the procedures are delegated to someone else. I conduct random quality checks regardless of how long a health professional has been performing the procedures in my practice. For example, I could have a P.A. who is very experienced and working under my supervision for more than 5 years and I would still maintain the same level of oversight and supervision. At unannounced times, I will walk into the room and watch the P.A. do a procedure that she may have performed thousands of times, just to make sure that she is maintaining proper technique and not getting sloppy or developing bad habits.

If you expect the worst, then it won't happen. It's inevitable that the unprepared have the worst disasters happen to them. In the case of the 20-something year old in Virginia who died because of lidocaine toxicity (overdosage of the topical anesthetic absorbed into his body) from application of a topical anesthetic cream prior to laser hair removal, his life may have been saved if proper measures had been taken. There are usually obvious signs of developing lidocaine toxicity (early signs can be lightheadedness, dizziness, ringing in the ears, difficulty breathing, anxiety) which if caught and recognized by a physician trained in proper cardiac and life resuscitation measures, would trigger the implementation of proper resuscitary measures that could save the patient's life. However, if there was not a physician on site and the nurse was not familiar with recognizing the symptoms and not able to administer proper emergency care, the patient may die before the local emergency room is contacted and the paramedics arrive on the scene.

There was a recently well published tragic event that involved a young female college student in North Carolina who was told to apply the topical anesthetic cream at home to her legs prior to going for laser hair removal at a plastic surgeon's laser clinic. She was found in her car dead at the side of the road with saran wrap covering both her legs. The saran wrap was used to help occlude the topical anesthetic cream in order to help the cream penetrate better into the skin. She may have had the cream on for hours.

Just looking at this case from a distance, I suspect that she did not know that applying a topical anesthetic cream to such a large surface area (both legs) under saran wrap occlusion can be quite dangerous if the cream is left on too long. She may have thought that the longer she left it on, the better the anesthetic effects, but without taking into consideration the possibility of lidocaine toxicity. Most of the cases of death related to lidocaine toxicity have involved usage of saran wrap for occlusion of the skin in order to aid in penetration.

One of the major complaints about topical anesthesia is that it takes so long to take effect and sometimes doesn't help take away the pain associated with laser procedures due to poor penetration of the active substance. The most common ingredients used are lidocaine, betacaine, and tetracaine. Lidocaine is the most common cause of toxicity. All ingredients may be associated with allergic reactions.

It usually takes about 1 to 2 hours of applying a topical anesthetic comprised of lidocaine 5% (i.e.: EMLA and Ela-Max/LMX are some brand names) under occlusion to achieve maximum anesthetic effects. This may not cause significant lidocaine absorption if a small surface area such as the upper lip or lower face were being treated. But when treating large surface areas such as the back or both legs, the amount of lidocaine that can be absorbed if a thick layer of the cream is applied under occlusion can be quite significant, and may even result in toxic or lethal amounts. The amount of lidocaine absorbed in the body is directly proportional to the amount applied and the length of time the cream is left on. Add an occlusive barrier such as saran wrap and the amount of lidocaine absorbed can be exponentially high.

In my practice, I use a topical compound using lidocaine and betacaine and tetracaine. There are several reasons I use this compound: (1) Faster onset of activity—it reaches maximum effect within 20 to 30 minutes instead of an hour with the anesthetics containing only lidocaine, (2) Better pain relief—the compounded anesthetic is 2 to 3 times more effective at 30 minutes than the lidocaine compounds are at 1 hour, (3) No need to use saran wrap for occlusion because of the better efficacy, thus keeping the level of anesthetic absorbed at a minimum. I conducted a comparison study between the triple anesthetic cream vs. EMLA vs. Ela-Max, which was published in Cosmetic Dermatology (Lee MWC. "Topical Triple-Anesthetic Gel Compared with 3 Topical Anesthetics." *Cosmetic Dermatology*. 2003;16:35-38).

The triple anesthetic cream should not be used in individuals who have allergies to any of those ingredients or to sulfa medications.

By keeping the exposure time to a minimum and not using occlusive saran wrap, the amount of anesthetic absorbed is kept to a minimum therefore decreasing the risk of lidocaine toxicity.

I also make sure that when we are treating large areas such as the back that we apply the topical anesthetic in quadrants or segments. For example, we separate the back into 6 different quadrants and apply the triple anesthetic cream to one quadrant at a time. We wipe the topical anesthetic cream prior to laser treatment of that quadrant, while at the same time applying topical anesthetic to another quadrant which will be properly anesthetized by the time we're done treating the first quadrant. We continue to wipe off cream and treat that quadrant while anesthetizing another quadrant. This keeps the amount of exposure to topical anesthesia to a safe amount. Also, we never apply saran wrap for occlusion since we're using the triple anesthetic cream.

I believe that in the case of the college student who died from lidocaine toxicity on her way to the North Carolina laser clinic, that several things would have changed her outcome. First, I believe it's unsafe practice to allow a patient to apply the topical anesthetic cream on their own at home. If she had an extreme reaction to the cream, there is no one to administer proper aid. The cream should only be applied in the physician's office under proper supervision and with access to the proper emergency equipment. Second, even if the cream were applied in the laser clinic, there still may have been problems. If she had a life-threatening reaction, the staff may not have been trained to recognize the symptoms and may not know how to administer proper emergency life-saving measures. The physician was not even on site at the clinic so if there were an emergency occurring there, the physician would not have been available to administer proper care. And with life-threatening events, there is no time to track down the physician and wait for them to arrive.

Another young woman died from similar causes in Arizona. There are many unfortunate cases of death resulting from lidocaine toxicity or allergic reactions to topical anesthetics. Many of these cases may have been prevented if proper safety precautions had been taken and if proper emergency measures had taken place within a certain narrow window of opportunity.

In my practice, I perform all the complicated laser treatments especially those involving intricate work around the eyes and face. I never let anyone else treat the eye area. I delegate certain treatments such as laser hair removal, acne laser and light treatments, photorejuvenation, microdermabrasion and light glycolic peels to a P.A. or R.N. I perform all other cosmetic procedures such as facial laser rejuvenation, laser skin resurfacing, leg vein treatments, Botox and filler injections (i.e., Collagen, Cosmoderm®/Cosmoplast®, Restylane®, Perlane®, Sculptra®, Hylaform®, Captique®).

Choosing the right doctor is the most important decision in the laser treatment process. If you go to an individual who is unethical enough to lie about their background and training, God knows what else they're willing to lie about and you don't want someone cutting corners when it comes to your health and well-being. Most important, remember that laser procedures are a MEDICAL procedure. These are not foo-foo cosmetic treatments like going for a facial or manicure. Major complications can and do occur. These are much less likely to ever occur if you are getting your treatment done by a qualified and competent physician's office. Some complications are inevitable (i.e., allergic reactions) so you'd much rather they happen while in the presence of a competent physician who knows how to deal with the problem rather than a huckster who wouldn't know what to do with a complication. It can make the difference between life and death. In a good doctor's care, laser treatments can produce wonderful results and are very safe. In an unqualified doctor's care, at best you may waste your money because they don't really know what they're doing so they can't recommend or offer the best treatments. They may appear cheaper but you get what you pay for. For example, some patients shop around based on price and they'll go to the clinic that offers FotoFacials at the lowest price but they don't properly inform you that it doesn't remove wrinkles and many of the larger and deeper blood vessels and pigmented lesions won't be gone especially those around the nose and let's suppose that's what you really wanted treated. They didn't properly educate you on the treatment options that would help you accomplish this. So they sign you up for a series of FotoFacials and even if they're cheaper, you find out at the end that you completely wasted your money after you go to a proper laser surgeon's office who informs you that wasn't the right procedure for your problems so you end up spending even more in the end to get it done right. So you're lucky if all you did was lose some money without getting good results. At worst, you may end up getting burned, scarred and permanently disfigured. Or even worse, dead.

I've heard a number of people, including doctors, say, "What's the big deal? It's not like it's brain surgery." Well, I wouldn't want them performing brain surgery on me either with that kind of attitude. It's that kind of lackadaisical attitude that has caused the public to not take cosmetic procedures seriously and which lures them into dangerous situations. It wasn't until after I finished my fellowship training that I had an entirely different outlook on the complexities and challenges of laser and cosmetic surgery and realized how ignorant I had been before. Ignorance allows one to trivialize any subject. I hadn't realized how much could go wrong until after I witnessed all the complications that got referred to UCSF during my fellowship. You learn the most from other people's mistakes. Anyone who claims that lasers are simple and doesn't require special training is displaying their profound ignorance.

Even if a poorly trained practitioner didn't actually maim someone with a laser, isn't it equally wrong for them to be denying the patient an opportunity to have the optimal treatment that only a true laser expert could provide them? Would you deny your patient the right to having a qualified cardiologist evaluate and treat a heart condition? One could argue that even if a family practitioner didn't cause direct immediate damage to the patient, that he may have prevented the patient from having a better quality life by not referring the patient to a qualified cardiologist for optimization of cardiac care. It's unethical for a family practitioner to provide substandard cardiac care and not refer to a qualified cardiologist. It's equally unethical for an untrained physician to provide substandard laser care and not refer to a qualified laser surgeon.

The hallmark of a bad family practitioner or GP is one who does not refer appropriately when necessary. If there's someone else better trained to perform a procedure, then the primary care physician should refer. They are preventing their patients from seeking optimal laser care by falsely presenting themselves as being adequately trained to perform laser treatments and not referring them to the laser specialists. One could argue that if you were in the middle of Wyoming and there were no other specialists other than family practitioners performing lasers, then your only choice is to see that doctor. But in a large metropolitan area with so many doctors board-certified in dermatology and fellowship-trained in laser and cosmetic surgery, there is no excuse for a primary care physician not to refer.

There are many places performing laser and cosmetic procedures illegally. Many people know of these places and are reluctant to step forward. You can and should report these operations to the authorities and the California Medical Board. By doing your civic duty, you could be saving a life.

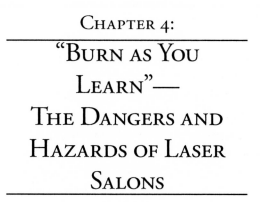

CHAPTER 4

"Burn as You Learn"— The Dangers and Hazards of Laser Salons

ONE OF THE BIGGEST issues regarding lasers is who gets to use the laser? This varies greatly state by state. Some states have absolutely no regulations at all—in these states, electrologists, beauticians, and even lay persons are legally performing laser procedures. It would be no surprise that surveys on this subject show that most physicians feel that they should maintain control of the device, and some non-physicians have stated that they are qualified to own and operate lasers.[1]

Beauticians, cosmetologists, aestheticians, hair stylists, tattoo artists, electrologists, and lay persons are buying lasers and then advertising for their services. There are no legal requirements for training, no quality control measures, no official quality standards or guidelines.

Most states have laws prohibiting the use of lasers by nonlicensed health professionals. The laws usually require that a laser can only be used by a physician or an appropriate licensed health professional (R.N., N.P., P.A.) who is properly supervised by a physician. However, there are major problems with enforcement of these laws. The lack of enforcement of existent laws governing proper laser usage and the subsequent need for the consumer to be educated for self-protection is the major impetus behind this chapter. There are many good laws that exist for the purpose of protecting the consumer from dangerous procedures. The consumer needs to be aware that the government agencies that should be enforcing these laws have not been doing their jobs. The consumer should not assume that Big Brother is looking out after him. So the consumer needs to be educated about the dangers and hazards that result from the improper usage of lasers by untrained and unqualified personnel and poorly operated salons. Consumers need to protect themselves from harm since the government is not cracking down on illegal activities and shutting these places down.

There is a great lack but vital need for extensive scientific evaluation of all laser systems, objective and reliable marketing by laser manufacturers, established training guidelines for laser operators, and legislation which restricts the use of lasers to physicians alone or strict guidelines on what constitutes proper physician supervision, and enforcement of the laws.

The FDA classifies lasers as prescriptive devices which by law can only be sold to physicians. The FDA requires that laser companies keep a registry of laser owners and that they keep track of what happens to these lasers. There are a number of doctors who buy lasers and sell them to nurses or aestheticians. Unfortunately, laser companies don't seem to be keeping track of what happens to the lasers that are sold because many of them end up in the secondary market which are then sold to nonphysicians. For example, a doctor may use a laser for a year and then decides he wants to sell it. He sells it to UsedLasers.com (made-up name), which is a clearinghouse for used lasers. This company doesn't care who buys the lasers as long as they have good credit. My grandmother could purchase a laser online from that company using a credit card. And no, my grandmother is not a physician.

Laser cosmetic surgery is a relatively new frontier that has gone through a tremendous boom in the last few years. It is common to open any newspaper in any major city in the U.S. and see dozens of ads for laser hair removal treatments being done in laser salons and spas. Laser salons are appearing in shopping malls across the U.S. almost as quickly as fast-food restaurants.

There's a combination of forces working together to create the current situation, which I would describe as the "Wild Wild West". Physicians who work in hospitals and medical groups taking insurance are tired of the low reimbursement rates and looking for additional income sources. The thought of cash paying procedures is very alluring to physicians. Laser companies are driven by selling lasers, the more they sell the better for their profit-earnings. There is an increasing lure for investors and entrepreneurs to cash in on the booming cosmetic laser industry by investing in laser spa/salon chains across the country. The market ultimately is driven by the incessant demand of consumers for anti-aging treatments and the desire to look younger and more beautiful.

The investors in laser chains will buy into franchises that promise big returns on their investment dollars, claiming there are limitless opportunities to capitalize on the $14 billion-plus cosmetic and laser industry. The franchising corporations will get a large group of investors to finance a chain of multiple laser salons located in many cities in various states across the country. The laser salons are positioned within shopping malls with high visibility and foot-traffic. The franchising corporation will usually strike up a deal with a laser company that gives them the best deal for purchasing mass quantities of lasers for their franchises. It's more cost efficient for them to purchase all their lasers with one company, so they will usually only offer one brand of laser. Each franchise will have the same lasers and offer the same procedures.

The franchising corporation will tell investors that they don't need to worry about not being physicians, that they can easily hire doctors to act as medical director of their laser salon. There is an endless supply of doctors who are sick and tired of dealing with insurance companies and eager for moonlighting opportunities. They approach doctors with an attractive arrangement—the doctor can earn money without even physically being present at the laser salon. The doctor may only have to be present one day a week or less and still get paid for the other days that he's not present but is "supervising" off-site. The doctor likes the idea of not having to deal with actually doing laser procedures he or she isn't qualified or trained to do because the franchising corporation promises to have nurses do all the work and they will be responsible for "training" the nurses. The doctors don't even have to know anything about the procedures. They are being used only to create a façade of legitimacy. If there really was need for a doctor, the client would truly be in trouble because the "supervising" doctor is usually an internist, family practitioner, general practitioner, emergency room physician, etc. who is not formally trained in cosmetic laser surgery or in skin care.

The modus operandi of these laser salons usually involves nurses doing all the evaluations and laser treatments. Only rarely is the doctor required to be present—in some cases, the doctor will give the Botox and Restylane injections. But often, all the procedures, lasers and injectables, are administered by the nurses. In some cases, there are no licensed health professionals doing any of the treatments or evaluations. They are being performed by aestheticians, cosmetologists, or laypersons.

It is considered the illegal practice of medicine in California and most other states for an aesthetician to perform lasers and inject Botox, Restylane and other fillers. It is illegal for a nurse to perform these procedures without the proper supervision of a physician.

The California Board of Nursing and the California Medical Board state that it is improper for a nurse to perform medical procedures (i.e.: lasers, Botox and filler injections) in a shopping mall or salon. These are not considered health care settings.

Nurses performing medical procedures in beauty salons, tattoo parlors, franchising salons and spas in shopping malls are in violation of California Medical Practices Act and Business and Professions Codes. According to **npr-b-5 (revised, Business and Professions Code 2725, Nursing Practice Act and California Code of Regulations 1474, Standardized Procedure Guidelines** (Board of Registered Nursing), "Beauty salons, health spas, shopping malls, and private residences do not meet the requirement of an organized health care system for the performance of standardized procedures." In other words, nurses cannot perform laser treatments in malls.

Laser hair removal and laser therapy are medical procedures that may be performed by a registered nurse under the direction of a physician only if the nurse is following a "standardized procedure"—a standardized procedure can only be done in a medical facility or hospital, not in a shopping mall.

Laypersons and nonphysicians invest in laser franchises and "rent" doctors and nurses to work for them. Often, the doctors and nurses become investors in the franchise as well. The doctor is present infrequently and the nurse does all the treatments. The doctor is paid to be a "medical director" of the franchise or "Doc-in-the-box". The entrepreneurs behind these franchises want to build a high-volume chain with each franchise appearing identical and supposedly delivering identical services with a drive-through mentality modeled after fast-food chains such as McDonald's. This is the "McLaser" paradigm.

"McLaser" franchises initially work because of discounting prices to try to get volume. The laser companies try to sell the owners of the franchise by promising to train their staff if they buy their lasers. It is illegal for laser companies to be involved with the "training" of physicians—training doctors and medical staff is the practice of medicine and can only be done by physicians in a health care setting or an institutionalized setting that is credentialed for training (i.e., universities and academic centers). "McLaser" tries to lowball everyone to get customers in. However, this quickly backfires because there are no discounts in costs or materials (i.e., McLaser has to pay the same price for the cost of Botox). So eventually they go out of business because they're not able to generate enough profit. They have high volume but low profit margins. In fact, many of these businesses hemorrhage money.

So why bother to shut them down if they eventually go out of business anyway? Because there's a sucker born every minute to replace them. Every time a laser chain closes down, several more open up in its place because they somehow think they're going to succeed where the previous one failed. It always follows the same pattern. Customers pay upfront for a discounted package deal—the owners initially are cash flush and ecstatic to see all the capital. Once they have to start honoring these package deals and perform the treatments with their costs being the same, they soon realize they can't afford to stay in business by offering such low prices. Just when the first lawsuits start pouring in, they close down leaving their customers with unfinished package deals and many people harmed, both physically and financially. They leave a blaze of victims in their wake.

Another thing that these franchises never take into account is that medical treatments by their very nature cannot be "mass-produced". Especially cosmetic procedures. Each laser treatment has to be customized to the individual's needs. There are no two people who can be treated in the exact same way (except perhaps twins—even then, they may have different needs and concerns which would require altering the treatments). The laser treatment is only as good as the physician's ability to properly and accurately diagnose the condition and recommend the correct treatment plan. The "McLaser" method of trying to fit everyone into the same cookie-cutter approach will inevitably result in some people having subpar treatments with no results and other people with overly aggressive treatments with severe complications. An experienced physician would be able to recognize those patients who had more sensitive skin who needed a more conservative approach and be able to recognize patients who may not be good candidates or unresponsive to treatments.

Laser salons lure patrons in by the promise of cheap deals and quick "lunch-hour" surgery, the use of loyalty cards and discount vouchers to encourage men and women to do repeat business, and an aggressive marketing and business strategy aimed at convincing customers to undergo costly and often unnecessary treatments.

Go to these places if you want to throw away your hard-earned money and support an industry that is harming people. Laser companies are in the business of making money. They are not in the business of training doctors or nurses to use lasers. The industry is driven by companies wanting to expand their market share. It started with laser companies recognizing that they could not survive by just selling to qualified doctors so they started selling to any doctor. But then they got even more greedy and wanted to expand into the salon/spa market because the doctor market got saturated. There are only so many doctors in the U.S. But if you expand beyond the physician market to lay persons, the market becomes infinitely bigger.

Laser companies use prominent dermatologists specializing in lasers to perform research and make the laser and procedures using that laser legitimate and accepted amongst the medical community. Once the laser and procedure have been accepted by dermatologists and plastic surgeons as safe and effective, the company then tries to expand their market by selling to nonaesthetic specialists such as family practitioners, internists, OB/Gyn's, emergency room physicians, etc. Having saturated the M.D. market, the companies then turned to dentists, chiropractors, podiatrists, optometrists, and even veterinarians. The laser company sales rep will approach an OB/Gyn and show them how much more money they could make if they started doing cosmetic laser procedures instead of practicing medicine involving insurance. They'll show them a business plan and promise to help them with advertising and marketing. The company will even promise to train the doctor and their staff to perform laser procedures. This usually involves sending them to a weekend course or seminar. Then the OB/Gyn will start using the laser in their practice, thinking this is all the training they need.

The laser company will tell the OB/Gyn that they have a built-in patient base upon which to market the laser procedures because they have all their medical patients that they can "convert" to cosmetic patients. They tell the OB/Gyn that since their patients trust them as their physician, they'll believe anything they tell them, so if they tell the patient that they're the best to perform laser hair removal on them, their trusting patients will believe them.

The laser company then approaches entrepreneurs interested in starting large laser cosmetic chains across the country and strike up a deal to sell them all the devices they need, help them with advertising and marketing, and also help "train" their staff. Once again, this bogus training consists of a weekend course or seminar, sometimes even less. They'll receive an instruction manual with some treatment settings and think that they can use these settings on everyone. They are completely incapable of dealing with any potential complications and they're not even aware that they can happen.

The vast majority of lasers are being sold to physicians and non-physicians who have no training in diagnosis of skin problems, and no training or knowledge of the myriad of complications that can occur with the skin or how to treat it. More than 75% of one laser company's sales have been to salons and spas.

Shareholders of laser companies that predominantly do business with nonphysicians and salons/spas need to be aware that they are at high risk of long-term complications and need to closely inspect the prospectus of these companies to see if the short-term gains come from risky deal-making. Common sense would dictate that it doesn't make good business sense to sell devices to those who aren't properly trained to use those devices. And as more states wake up and realize the extent of the problems wrought by this technology and realize their laws have not caught up to the current state of the technology, they will pass more laws and regulations governing laser usage and many of these laser companies will be involved with illegal use of their devices. As it stands, many laser companies are in violation of state and federal laws by selling to nonphysicians. Even if a particular state doesn't regulate the usage of lasers, companies that sell laser devices to nonphysicians are violating the FDA rules that govern sale of lasers only to physicians.

According to the FDA, manufacturers are required to track certain devices from their manufacture through the distribution chain when they receive an order from the agency to implement a tracking system for a certain type of device. The purpose of the device tracking is to ensure that manufacturers of certain devices establish tracking systems that will enable them to promptly locate devices in commercial distribution. Tracking information may be used to facilitate notifications and recalls ordered by FDA in the case of serious risks to health presented by the devices.

Manufacturers must adopt a method of tracking devices whose failure would be reasonably likely to have serious, adverse health consequences. The necessity of tracking lasers, as a prescriptive device, makes sense given that a malfunction in any laser device could present serious health risks. Presumably, one should be able to call any laser company and track the whereabouts of any device.

The Center for Devices and Radiological Health of the FDA has classified intense pulsed light and some laser devices as Class II prescriptive devices and other laser devices as Class III devices. Class II intense pulsed light/laser devices or Class III laser devices per FDA requirements are sold to physicians only and are considered prescriptive devices. Further information regarding FDA requirements may be found at www.fda.gov.

In any and every state, a non-medically licensed layperson owning a light or laser device would be in violation of FDA guidelines. In many states, it is required that only a physician can own a laser.

In California, an example of an illegal business would be a chain of laser salons that is owned by a nonphysician that hires a physician to be a "medical director" of the chain and pays that physician a salary to be on staff. The chain and the lasers are owned by the corporate entity. By law in California, a physician cannot partner with a nonlicensed medical practitioner to form a corporation that would own a laser.

I often read on website chat rooms that people think the laser salons and spas are good for driving down laser prices that are perceived to be too high. It is unfortunate that people would have any good associations with these enterprises. The prices of laser treatments are driven by the actual cost of the equipment. Businesses that undercharge in order to capture market share will not be able to stay in business for long, and by supporting these businesses, you're hurting legitimate businesses that are charging appropriate prices. The businesses that undercharge go out of business and take your money with them because most likely they charged for prepaid packages upfront, realize they can't charge such low prices and stay in business, close down, and run off with your money before you're able to get all your treatments.

I often hear of people bragging that they personally never got harmed (yet!) at a laser salon or spa. That may be true, but these people are supporting an industry that is harming many others. By supporting these fringe businesses, they are aiding and abetting in their crimes. They are enabling them to continue their reckless endangerment of the public. And given enough time, they will leave a blaze of harmed individuals behind.

There was a laser hair removal chain in California called Nuvo International. They were based in Las Vegas, Nevada, and owned by

Jeff Schmidt and his wife, Bonnie Schmidt, R.N., Chris Pederson, M.D., and Norm Valiene. At their peak in 2005 they had 41 salons in California, Oregon, and Washington.

They created and formed franchising opportunities—opening locations in Nevada, Washington, Oregon, and California. They sold franchises to nonphysicians and purchased lasers for use in the various franchises. In doing so, they violated various state laws and FDA regulations. These include *Title 21 of the United States Code, FDA Reg. 800 ET seq.* Under both federal and California statutes and regulations, laser hair removal devices are categorized as prescriptive or dangerous devices and sales of such prescriptive or dangerous devices and sales are restricted to licensed physicians. The lasers/IPL devices purchased by Nuvo are classified under federal law as **prescriptive devices** (21 CFR 801.109). Federal law specifically forbids the distribution of prescriptive devices (lasers/IPL) to laypersons without a prescription. This means that Nuvo International cannot own/possess/control a prescriptive device because it is not a physician or a medical corporation.

California Health and Safety Code 111440-111470 regulates the ownership/distribution of dangerous (prescriptive) devices—stating that it is illegal to sell to a layperson or for a layperson to purchase/own a laser/IPL.

Business and Professions Code 2406 states that medical corporations in California must be physician owned (51%) with all other shareholders holding medical licensure in California. Nuvo owned at least 51% of each of the local Nuvo franchises, with many of the sites having additional shareholders that were either entirely or partially made up of laypersons. A lay (unlicensed) person cannot own any shares of a medical corporation or practice. A physician cannot partner with a layperson in forming a medical corporation or a medspa.

Starting a franchise usually involves considerable capital investment. The reason that many physicians are partnering with laypersons in forming medspas and laser salons is because they need the capital investment and a larger pool to share the financial risk, and in order to raise enough capital had to expand their investment portfolio to include laypersons.

Unlike McDonald's, which can have comparable food and service at each franchise by following their formula, "McLaser" cannot reproduce the same results between each franchise. The nurses hired to perform treatments are so variable in their backgrounds and most lack even the slightest hint of training. They receive some rudimentary instruction (one or 2 days) and are told to refer to a company treatment manual, which is like giving a user's manual to a person who has never driven a car before and telling them to use the manual in order to figure out how to drive.

On a website, a Nuvo employee revealed that the company's motto was "Burn as You Learn." This employee said that the company hired nurses and staff without any training and often would not even bother to provide the barest bones of training, not even sending them to a weekend course. The nurses would literally learn as they went along, learning from their mistakes. They would "burn as they learned". After burning a patient, they may conclude that was a reasonable outcome and think that it was normal for patients to experience burns—that it came with the territory.

Many patients began to come forward after suffering permanent scarring and disfigurements. Nuvo's supervising physicians were overseeing multiple facilities. In many instances they would only show up for an hour or two, once or twice a month. The physicians employed by Nuvo have specialties that include Colon & Rectal Surgery, none appear to be dermatologists.

Under the threat of mounting lawsuits and financial malfeasance by Nuvo directors, Nuvo filed chapter 11 bankruptcy in Nevada. This action prevented any of the malpractice and personal injury lawsuits from progressing.

Nuvo's assets were sold to Goldin Capital Management, which reopened all Nuvo locations under the name "MedSpa". Goldin changed names of "MedSpa" to "Lumity". They continue to operate in the same locations and in the same manner as Nuvo. This is a "slight of hand" that frequently occurs when one illegal business closes down only to be replaced by a similar one with a different name.

There continue to be a steady stream of patients who have been harmed by unsupervised and untrained personnel at "medspas" such as Nuvo and others. Throughout the nation, other examples are reported. Incidences of death from topical anesthetic (numbing) creams applied before laser hair removal treatments are reported. In Florida, a fake Botox scandal surfaces with multiple injuries and the ominous release that over 220 centers throughout the U.S. have been using the non-FDA approved fake Botox without disclosing this to their patients. Cases of illegal Silicone injections, fake plastic surgeons, backroom surgery in salons flourish. Other noted cases include the Greenhouse Day Spa in Manhattan burning a woman with a laser by a treatment from a cosmetologist, and the deaths by lidocaine toxicity that occurred in Arizona and North Carolina. There is also the case of Danny Faiello, an electrologist posing as a doctor in Manhattan who accidentally killed a woman during a cosmetic procedure and then buried her body in his garage.

Laser companies that sell lasers to nonphysicians are also violating federal laws. This has become prevalent in the industry. Because one laser company has done so, other laser manufacturers follow suit. They will continue to do so until the FDA and other governmental agencies that should be monitoring their activities start enforcing the laws.

The weekend warriors who attend weekend seminars on laser cosmetic surgery and emerge with self-designated titles such as "laser cosmetic aesthetician" and "director of laser and cosmetic surgery at the Rejuvenation Center of Anytown, USA." The Mount Cordoba Medical Center Laser Center (not real name) is run by an R.N. named Shelley (not her real name) who is the "laser cosmetic specialist" who administers all the laser treatments without any physician supervision. Doctors who are members of the medical center refer all patients to this laser center because they get a percentage of all their referrals (a referral fee). They charge outrageously low prices on laser procedures—patients go there and are never told that they will be treated by a nurse, they never even meet a doctor. One patient came to me with white scars on her face, arms, and legs because Shelley treated her cherry angiomas with the "FotoFacial" which is an intense pulsed light device that is inappropriate to be treating cherry angiomas. Cherry angiomas are small tiny discrete red spots which need a higher intensity laser with a smaller spot size capable of treating such small discrete spots—the intense pulsed light handpiece is a large rectangle which is not capable of delivering a focused beam of light without affecting surrounding skin (a cherry angioma is usually 1-2 mm, the handpiece of the intense pulsed light is at least 5-10 mm in diameter which affects the skin surrounding the cherry angioma which can result in blistering or damage to the surrounding skin causing hypopigmentation).

The "zebra-stripes" caused by IPL devices have become a common adverse effect associated with those treatments. I see all sorts of patients with strange linear, rectangular, circular, or other unnatural geometric shapes imprinted on their skin by practitioners not properly trained to operate lasers.

These salons come and go but they leave a blaze of victims in their wake—harmed financially and physically. As if it weren't bad enough to get physically burned and scarred, it's even worse to realize that you paid good money to have that done. After seeing so many complications, it leaves one to ponder that the only thing sinful about the need to have cosmetic surgery for vanity is to not have it done right, and to do it on the cheap.

And the prepaid hair removal package—the money disappears but the hair remains.

Salons and lower end laser clinics may charge extremely low prices for laser hair removal. Ads that offer "laser hair removal for $99" draw people in the door. They are offered prepaid packages of 3-6 treatments that they pay for in advance. After 3 treatments, they'll find that they need more treatments that they were not told up front about and then get hit up for more money. Oftentimes these salons are low-balling the prices so much that they can't stay in business and end up closing their doors with many patients who are left hanging with unfinished prepaid treatments remaining in their package deal and have no recourse. Money gone but hair remains. Bankrupt businesses do not have to settle their accounts.

Worse yet than losing your money, you may be left with mutilating scars and disfigurements that can never be removed. It's not like buying a discounted TV that you can return if you find out it's defective. This is your body and health that you're experimenting with and trying to cut corners with. You get one body and there are no guarantees or exchanges allowed.

Always remember: you get what you pay for. And if you can't afford to get it done right, don't do it at all. It will cost many times more to fix the damage (if indeed it can be fixed at all). And finally, if it sounds to good to be true, it probably is.

If 5 different doctors tell you one thing, and then some strip mall salon tells you another, who are you going to believe? If the salon or practitioner tells you that they'll be able to remove hairs 100% completely with only 3 treatments, they're lying!

The sad part about bargain shopping for cosmetic laser treatments is that in the end, you don't really end up saving money. You find out that you would have paid approximately the same in the long run if you'd seen a legitimate laser expert in a real medical setting but that the difference is the legitimate laser expert told you the truth upfront, you just chose to believe the lies that the laser salon told you, thinking you could get a real bargain. And even if you did save 50%--what kind of deal is to get a substandard treatment at 50% off? If you were going for LASIK eye surgery, would you think it's a good deal to get only partial vision correction for half the price?

Most of the dangers and problems with nonphysicians practicing medicine are immediately obvious. Corporations are not licensed to practice medicine and most states clearly define it as illegal for them to either partner with or control physicians' decision-making abilities. Besides the blatant examples of scarring, burning, and disfigurement, other dangers lurk when nonphysicians or non-qualified physicians perform laser treatments. Only dermatologists are trained specifically to recognize and treat skin conditions. It is unreasonable to expect that anyone else could competently spot and treat appropriately melanoma and other skin cancers. Incidences of skin cancers being "treated" with lasers (because they were misdiagnosed as benign skin lesions) have been reported. Also because of the high variability of response that individuals have to any treatments, the ability to understand the science of the skin when treating with a laser is essential. Melding the ability and training to understand the body's largest organ (the skin) with the skills and qualifications to operate a laser is quite rare. Having the knowledge on how to devise proper treatment parameters goes beyond even what dermatologists receive in their residency programs. Money has clouded the judgment of many and has made many risk the safety of their patients.

The slippery slope of illegal activity has started. It started with physicians who did not properly supervise procedures and followed with physicians who were not trained or qualified entering the field. Their lack of knowledge and training encourage nonphysician staff (who in many instances knew more about the procedures than the doctor) to believe that they were qualified to perform these same procedures on their own in the context of their own business. Unscrupulous manufacturers and carpet bagging physicians pushed and promoted the business of "cosmetic" medicine to all who would listen. When competition and sales tightened, they hit the nonphysician market with total abandon—patient consequences and the law be damned. Nonphysicians, lured by a market that they previously thought off limits rushed in without evaluating the ethical considerations. Many, knowing that they were already skirting proper conduct and violating legal guidelines, ventured into outright illegality in order to prosper. Case after case has come forward of people being victimized by the injections of dangerous, non-FDA approved substances, permanent scarring from botched treatments, crippling pain following substandard care, and in some instances death. All of this continues unabated with laissez-fair attitude of the governing medical boards, politicians, and professional societies.

What can the public do to protect themselves? (because no one is going to do it for you!)

1. Only go to a facility run by a physician **board-certified in dermatology** where the physician is on-site and evaluates you before any procedure is performed and will make the decisions regarding treatment.

    You can find out if a dermatologist (or any other physician) is board-certified by contacting the American Board of Medical Specialties. Their website is:

    www.abms.org

(One caveat: you have to register with the site to get a password.)

The American Academy of Dermatology and the American Society for Dermatologic Surgery are excellent resources for finding information on qualified dermatologists. The following online sites provide a directory of dermatologists:

www.asds-net.org
www.aad.org

One major caveat is that the AAD and ASDS, although highly regarded organizations, do not list whether a dermatologist is board-certified. But they're at least a good starting point.

2. Ask questions about the physician's qualifications—do not accept that the physician is "trained in treating the skin" or that they are a "skin expert". If they do not clearly state and put in writing that they are a board-certified dermatologist, then you can assume that they are not!

3. Ask about the physician's training in laser. Did they have formal training in lasers such as a fellowship? Or did they learn by attending weekend courses? If they had fellowship training in lasers, they would clearly state that and put it in writing. Do not accept a vague, "I have excellent training in lasers!" (Some doctors consider a weekend course 'excellent training'.) Or, "I've been doing lasers for years!" (They could have been doing it wrong for years!) Pin them down and ask exactly what kind of training that was. Find out if they are a "dabbler" or a trained laser practitioner specializing in lasers. Evidence of a dabbler would be doing lasers once a week or twice a month, renting lasers, owning only one laser and claiming it does everything, etc. A physician specializing in lasers would own many lasers and be doing many laser procedures everyday.

4. The ideal physician to perform laser treatments is a **board-certified dermatologist** who has **fellowship training** in lasers and cosmetic surgery.

Every board-certified dermatologist I know puts that designation on their business card, letterhead, stationery, advertisements, and all written materials. You don't need to ask if they are a board-certified dermatologist because it is prominently displayed on all their written materials and advertisements. A big red flag is a business card that says, "Skin

Specialist." You can bet that person is not a board-certified dermatologist, otherwise the card would say so.

I am truly annoyed by patients who come into my office and are provided with written information about my credentials and background prior to meeting me, and then actually ask me if I'm a board-certified dermatologist. That is a clear indication that they didn't even bother to read all the written information we provided them. This kind of person is just plain lazy and not taking their visit seriously. There are many good doctors with sterling qualifications who take the time to properly educate their patients and provide ample written materials about their credentials just as I do but who are nonetheless inundated with unnecessary questions on a daily basis. I am not telling you to badger the doctor unnecessarily. Doctors who are proud of their credentials will proudly display their training and credentials for you to see and this should be quite obvious to the observant patient.

The danger signs you need to be aware of are the doctors who do not clearly put in writing on their business card, letterhead, yellow pages, advertisements, website, and other written materials that they are a "board-certified dermatologist". If the business card says something like, "board-certified and specializing in dermatology and skin care," or "board-certified and skin specialist"—these statements are all suspect and you can assume they are not the genuine McCoy.

It's easy to do some background checking on the doctor even before you meet them. Read the website carefully for the essential details I mentioned above—ignore all the hype and advertising jargon about the "attentive staff and beautiful surroundings" and the other touchy-feely stuff. Get down to the nitty-gritty and find out who exactly is this doctor you're going to see and what are their credentials? Then cross-check them with other sources by doing an on-line search or by calling the American Medical Association and the State Medical Board to verify their credentials and training. The first thing I do when I encounter a physician advertisement or website is I look up their board-certification and specialty on the AMA website.

A physician misrepresenting their specialty to the public really should be subject to the same truth-in-advertising laws we impose on everything else. When a consumer buys a tomato, they expect to buy a tomato, not an orange. If the grocer bags 6 oranges instead of 6 tomatoes, you take them back and ask for a refund. It doesn't matter if the grocer insists they gave you tomatoes if they're really oranges. If the grocer says it doesn't matter, you'll most likely feel deceived and cheated. If a doctor advertises himself as a dermatologist, you expect to be seeing a dermatologist, not a radiologist. It would be fine for a radiologist to be performing laser treatments as long as they told you they were a radiologist, then you could make the decision knowing what their background and training is. And you may decide to let the radiologist treat you, especially if you lived in a rural area where there were no dermatologists. But you ultimately want to make the choice with full disclosure. How could you make an informed decision if you weren't even aware of the doctor's true specialty? The most sacred thing between a physician and patient is trust and honesty. If a doctor is willing to lie to you about their specialty, what else could they be lying about? Misrepresenting one's specialty is a major breach of trust and shows total lack of regard for the sacred physician-patient relationship.

I may decide to substitute an orange for a tomato in a recipe, but that's my choice. And I don't want to be deceived about what I'm getting. Patients have the right to the same with their doctors. They deserve to know what they're getting.

What bothers me most about the burgeoning popularity of laser and cosmetic treatments is not increased competition. As one doctor, I can only see so many patients. These other practitioners are not a threat to my business because I can only see so many patients in one day. What bothers me the most is seeing so many physicians turn themselves into salesmen and charlatans and turning their back on the honor code and abusing the trust they have with their patients to coerce them into doing laser and cosmetic treatments that they may not be adequately trained to perform, all for the sake of generating cash flow. A radiologist may justify keeping their "identity" hidden because they're afraid of not attracting patients to their new laser clinic. But that radiologist is starting down the slippery slope of creating mistrust that can never be rectified once lost. A patient should rightfully never trust anything else that physician ever told them if they found out that physician was misrepresenting their training and specialty. A radiologist making a patient think they are anything but a radiologist, even if it's only by omission of the truth, is actively engaged in deception and lying.

I would like to see legislation passed that would mandate that physicians are legally required to provide board-certification information to the public. I never used to believe this was necessary until now with the vast amount of misrepresentation occurring due to so many physicians wanting to jump on the laser and cosmetic bandwagon.

About 9 out of 10 laser ads that I see in the newspapers and on websites are for medical practices and laser salons employing physicians and nonphysicians who are not properly trained to perform lasers. That's quickly changing to being more like 99 out of 100 ads.

The media has presented over the past few years an increasing number of stories of botched-up cosmetic surgery being performed by nonphysicians and mistakenly treated them as if they were anecdotal occasional cases. They are not anecdotal, they were signs of the impending tidal wave that was about to hit, and now it's a category 5.

References

[1] Wagner RF Jr, Brown T, McCarthy EM, McCarthy RA, Uchida T. Dermatologist and electrologist perspectives on laser procedures by nonphysicians. Dermatologic Surgery. 2000 Aug; 26(8):723-7.

CHAPTER 5:

SHADOWS, ROGUES, AND DABBLERS

AFTER FINISHING MEDICAL SCHOOL training, I developed an interest in becoming an expert of the skin and decided to pursue residency training in dermatology. During my dermatology residency I became interested in skin cancer surgery and Mohs micrographic surgery and reconstruction. I was also fascinated with laser and cosmetic surgery and looked for ways to get additional training in these subspecialties. There are several fellowship programs that provide multidisciplinary training in these subspecialties. Some programs only provide training in Mohs micrographic surgery (the gold standard for skin cancer surgery) which allows the surgeon to map out the full extent of the skin cancer by looking at the tissue margins at the time of surgery so it eliminates the guess work and allows the surgeon to be able to pinpoint the exact location of the skin cancer and remove all the cancer cells. After removing the skin cancer, there needs to be reconstructive repair of the surgical defect left behind. Some programs only train the physician in Mohs and provide little training in reconstructive surgery. Graduates from these programs lack the ability to fix complex surgical wounds and often need to refer the closures to a plastic surgeon. Many people mistakenly think a plastic surgeon is the best person to remove a skin cancer because they're primarily consumed with the way they'll look afterwards. But a plastic surgeon can't guarantee that they were able to remove all the skin cancer so there's a much greater chance of recurrence. And if the skin cancer recurs, it oftentimes is much more aggressive and more difficult to remove without causing a greater disfigurement. The key with skin cancer is to remove it all and to remove it all the first time around. For skin cancers, there are 2 equally important concerns: (1) To remove all the skin cancer and (2) to maintain a normal appearance after the skin cancer removal. It doesn't matter how great the plastic surgeon makes you look afterwards if he doesn't remove the entire skin cancer. And many patients are unhappy with some Mohs surgeons who do not perform an adequate repair and leave a less than desirable cosmetic result.

The best Mohs fellowship programs provide excellent training in reconstructive surgery as well as Mohs micrographic surgery for removing skin cancers. The doctors graduating from these programs have expert training in removing the skin cancer and also ensuring that the cosmetic result will be the best possible.

Even fewer programs provide laser and cosmetic surgery training. And far fewer programs provide a combination of Mohs surgery, reconstructive surgery, and laser and cosmetic surgery program. One of these programs is at UCSF and I knew if I wanted to get the best training in this multidisciplinary field, that UCSF would be the top program to receive that training. I was extremely fortunate and privileged to have been accepted into this exceptional training program that would provide me with the best training in the world in the areas I wanted to specialize in: Mohs micrographic surgery, reconstructive surgery, dermatologic surgery, laser and cosmetic surgery. I knew that graduating from this program would allow me to practice in my chosen field with the best training possible and feel confident that I would be able to provide the best care possible to my patients.

I can honestly say that if I had not received the training that I did, that I would never have dreamed of performing the procedures that

I do. Having gone through a fellowship program, I had even greater respect for the type of complications that can occur. Even in the best hands, things can go wrong and it's absolutely essential that the physician know how to deal with these complications as they arise.

In the last several years I have seen an alarming increase in the number of physicians and even nonphysicians who are willing to put their patients at risk because they lack formal training to perform the procedures they do. These physicians did not pursue the proper training as I did but yet still try to perform the procedures that I do. It's unbelievable to see the number of internists, family practitioners, OB/Gyn's, general practitioners, anesthesiologists, radiologists, even psychiatrists and pediatricians, you name it, every specialist wants a piece of the action. And they're only doing it for money. They have absolutely no other rationale to be practicing out of the scope of their training and specialization other than to make an extra buck. And then there's the nurses, nurse practitioners, physician assistants, and cosmetologists/aestheticians who are performing procedures that they are not trained or licensed to perform. It is amazing for me to see how many health professionals are willing to throw away their sense of propriety and ethical conduct just to make money from procedures that aren't even necessary.

Cosmetic procedures by definition are medically unnecessary. Some people think they are frivolous and unnecessary or vain or indulgent. Other people think they can be life-changing and necessary and argue that in some cases they could be deemed necessary. No matter what you think of cosmetic and laser procedures, I think most people would agree that if you opt to get them done, you should at least go to someone who is qualified to perform them.

I am proud of my training and my specialty. I am grateful that I have the expertise, training, and skills to help people with cosmetic concerns look and feel the best about themselves. I am concerned that just because these procedures are "cosmetic" and therefore not life-threatening, that many people tend to trivialize them and put them in the category of facials and manicures. The fact that so many doctors and nurses who never received formal training in these procedures think that they can just go and practice on patients after attending a weekend course shows their lack of respect for cosmetic procedures and for the patients who seek them. I treat patients with cosmetic concerns with the same level of care and concern as I treat patients with medical conditions because the individual seeking care does not differentiate between the two. A person who is distressed about their wrinkles deserves the same respect and professionalism as a person who is distressed about their diabetes. Of course, insurance should pay for diabetes but not for anti-aging procedures but that shouldn't put the cosmetic patient in an inferior category. In other words, the cosmetic patient deserves to receive the same conditions and to receive the same considerations as a diabetic patient. I would never dare presume to treat a diabetic patient because that's not my specialty. I would refer the diabetic patient to an internist or endocrinologist to manage. So why does the internist or endocrinologist think they have the proper training and skills to treat a cosmetic patient?

It is exactly because of the payment set-up that lures physicians and nurses into this field. Diabetic patients are covered by insurance because it is a medical condition. Doctors no longer like taking insurance because the reimbursements from the insurance companies are inadequate. So they look at the cosmetic field as being very lucrative because cash-paying patients pay out-of-pocket for elective procedures. I did not go into this field to avoid dealing with insurance. I went into this field because I have a fascination with the subject and wanted to learn everything I could about it and receive the best training possible so that I could be the best at what I do. If I had a fascination with performing eye surgery with cutting-edge technology such as the LASIK procedure, I would have tried to get into the best ophthalmology residency program and then apply for the best oculoplastic surgery fellowship program.

During my internship year spent in OB/Gyn, I realized that this was not the right career choice for me. This was the impetus for my switching into dermatology. If I had decided to dedicate myself to a career in OB/Gyn, I can guarantee that it would never have dawned on me to perform cosmetic procedures that I wasn't formally trained in. I am astonished at the number of OB/Gyn's who are cutting down on the amount of OB/Gyn they practice and replacing it with cosmetic and laser procedures. The most egregious part of this is that there is a great need for OB/Gyn services. They are turning their back on the specialty they were trained to perform and for which there is a great need in exchange for performing services they have no formal training or expertise in. If they had such a burning desire to do cosmetic procedures, why didn't they pursue the proper training like I did?

How do any of these doctors who are not trained to perform cosmetic procedures justify doing them? These procedures are unnecessary so they can't argue that they're saving people's lives. Imagine what the medical profession and the public would say if suddenly all sorts of doctors not trained in neurosurgery all decided they wanted to do neurosurgery. Some may argue that cosmetic surgery is not neurosurgery. But then I go back to my other argument that cosmetic patients deserve to be treated with the same respect and professionalism as neurosurgery patients.

I have seen many doctors who have caused serious complications on their cosmetic patients due entirely to their lack of training who were quite cavalier in dealing with these complications. Their attitude was that these patients deserved what they got because they were so vain to begin with, and what are a few scars on the face anyway? It's not the end of the world, it's not like you're dead. And just be glad that you're not as sick as that neurosurgery patient. I have heard some doctors say the patient deserved what they got because they didn't do their due diligence in researching the doctor's background and find out that they're a colorectal surgeon and not a cosmetic surgeon or dermatologist —so if the patient couldn't take their own health care seriously, why should the doctor?

There are varying degrees of severity of professional transgressions in the field of cosmetic laser surgery. I've separated them into three main categories: Shadows, Rogues, and Dabblers.

"Shadows" are the practitioners who aid and abet in the illegal practice of medicine. Also known as absentee or phantom practitioners. They lurk in the background as sponsoring physicians or pseudomedical directors who run "Doc-in-the-Boxes". These are free-standing clinics or spas or salons in shopping malls which advertise laser services with a supposed "medical director" on staff. This doctor is usually a doctor licensed in internal medicine, family practice, emergency medicine, OB/Gyn or some other specialty not trained to perform cosmetic laser procedures. Many of these doctors are older retired physicians looking for moonlighting positions or doctors who are unhappy with their primary medical practice and looking for additional income. They are a front for lower level practitioners such as nurses, nurse practitioners, or physician assistants who are performing cosmetic and laser procedures without proper training or supervision. The appeal to these physicians is that they can run a side business outside of their normal practice, which brings in extra income without having to do any work. The "medical director" usually has a primary medical practice that they keep separate. Typical scenarios consist of the doctor showing up once a week or even less. The nurses perform the procedures without ever having the doctor present to evaluate the patient or treat or supervise. The doctor makes occasional appearances to give the clinic an air of legitimacy. The worst part is these "shadow practitioners" do not possess proper training or skills themselves so that even if there were complications, they wouldn't be of much help. It's like the blind leading the blind. The nurse is poorly trained and "supervised" by a physician who also lacks training.

"Rogues" are doctors and nurses who have absolutely no training in lasers and perform treatments on patients without any care as to the consequences. They know they are inadequately trained but that doesn't stop them from exposing their patients to unnecessary harm. It falls into the category of reckless endangerment. At worst the rogue doctors and nurses cause physical and emotional harm to the patient with complications such as burning, scarring, disfigurement, even death can ensue. At best, their actions may not result in physical harm but they do not provide the standard of care in delivering cosmetic services and treatments. They do not deliver what they promise and cause the consumer to lose faith because they've been sold a bill of goods that they could not deliver. In other words, they cause the patient to spend money under false pretenses—money that could have been put to better use, like going to a qualified cosmetic surgeon who could provide them with the proper treatment, instead of wasting hard-earned money on a charlatan.

Many rogue nurses and doctors are lured into the cosmetic field by promises of an easier lifestyle and easy money (not true—a false perception). They're tired of dealing with sick patients with real medical problems in the hospital. They're tired of caring for patients who have problems that they were trained to deal with. They want a change of pace and think that providing laser cosmetic services would provide them with the easy life. Rogue nurses wantonly go out on their own to start up their own laser clinic, thinking they want to be an entrepreneur and not have to answer to any doctors. Many rogue nurses started out working under the auspices of a shadow practitioner, a sponsoring doctor who's board-certified in internal medicine or other specialty not trained to perform cosmetic procedures. These nurses were never properly trained themselves and realize that their supervising physician is just as clueless in this field and so their "supervision" really is a joke. The nurses start thinking that the doctor doesn't add anything to the equation so why not go out on their own so they don't have to split any of the profits with the doctor. The nurses start thinking they're tired of making money for the doctor who really isn't doing anything except lending an air of legitimacy so they strike out on their own. The incompetence of the doctor enables the nurse to think that they're more capable than the doctor. Since the nurse is performing all the treatments without any real supervision or involvement from the doctor, the nurse (and the patients) begins to perceive that the doctor is unnecessary. Many of these nurses go out into the community and start up their own laser clinic. A common ploy is to "rent-a-doc" by paying a doctor a fee to lend their license to give the clinic an air of legitimacy. But this way the nurse is in control and calls the shots and the doctor isn't even pretending to be supervising. This is a variation of the shadow practitioner in which the doctor was the instigator and aided and abetted in the illegal practice of medicine by hiring and sponsoring nurses to work under them with the guise that the doctors were in charge and supervising. Rogue nurses decide to flip around the situation so that they're the owners of the clinic and use a "rent-a-doc" for the license only but the doctor has no other role.

Rogue doctors are physicians who have been trained in one field but decide that they want to disregard the Hippocratic oath and expose patients to unnecessary danger but practicing a specialty they weren't trained to perform. A pediatrician who decides to practice OB/Gyn would be a rogue doctor. A psychiatrist who decides to perform plastic surgery is a rogue doctor. They decide that they're tired of their dreary lives and wish they would have trained in a presumably more lucrative and less taxing field, but they don't want to go back to get the proper training. That would require applying to an appropriate residency and/or fellowship program to get the proper and necessary formal training to be competent in the field. But this would require too much time and work. They would rather shortcut the system and forego going through any training. Do not feel sorry for these doctors if they complain that they've always had a burning desire to perform facelifts instead of colonoscopies—there is a way for them to get the proper training, they're just plain LAZY.

It's egregious, unconscionable, and unethical for physicians and nurses who are well-trained and qualified to practice a certain field of medicine to turn their backs on the field they were trained to perform and jump ship to an entirely different field they're not even trained to perform. The worst part is that they're leaving behind gaps in the field they were trained to perform where there are great shortages. When residency programs are allotted a certain number of training slots each year, there is a lot of research that goes into determining what the public need is for each field. When physicians take up valuable spots in residency training programs and then later on do not continue to practice the specialty they were trained in, they leave big gaps behind. They should have let someone else take the spot if they weren't going to be committed to practicing it. That way they wouldn't be harming the public good by falsely creating the perception that there would be enough physicians in their specialty practicing. For example, if it's predetermined that the U.S. needs 100,000 internists and these spots are filled with residents who presumably will practice internal medicine but then a few years later it turns out that half of these internists decide to practice cosmetic laser surgery instead of practicing internal medicine, there will be huge problems with patients getting access to a primary care physician. Imagine the difficulty for patients accessing an internist because they've converted increasing parts of their practice to performing Botox and laser hair removal. And opening up a side business to increase revenue leads to the problems associated with improper supervision previously discussed.

And nurses who have a hankering for working in the cosmetic laser field should seek training and employment under a properly trained cosmetic laser expert and commit themselves to working under the supervision of this physician. They should resist the urge to go "do it on their own". If they truly desire complete autonomy then they should apply for medical school and go through the necessary training to become a physician who specializes in cosmetic laser surgery.

A nurse friend informed me that her colleague left a job working in the ICU to work for a laser clinic that was owned and run by non-physicians. There was no physician ever present. The nurse was "trained" by the owners. The "training" consisted of her receiving treatment on her own face. She had burns and scars on her neck resulting from the hair removal treatment. The owners just said, "That happens." And all the nurses at the laser clinic assumed that this was just an expected outcome from laser hair removal. She went on to burning many customers and just told them this was to be expected. She asked her friend to find out from me what I normally do for post-care after lasers. I thought it was strange when this nurse kept asking me about my post-laser protocol and was inquiring about what I would do for someone who was burned after a laser procedure. I told this nurse friend to inform her friend that she's working for an illegal clinic but that nurse continues to work there. Her friend informed me that two other nurses decided to quit after they felt they were being pushed to force clients to sign up for unnecessary procedures. She said the owners came in one day and said they weren't generating enough income and that they would have to double the number of procedures they were performing by making customers sign up for more procedures even if they didn't think they needed them. The people involved with this illegal laser clinic have absolutely no regard for the care or well-being of their clients. They're simply a money mill. Their clients consist largely of strippers, exotic dancers, and employees from local clubs and bars. They also take advantage of people who are less educated and don't speak English as their primary language.

"Dabblers" are doctors and nurses who don't really specialize in lasers but "dabble" in them. These may include dermatologists, plastic surgeons, otolaryngologists, and other surgical subspecialties that may have cosmetic training. They spend the majority of their time performing various cosmetic procedures but don't really have formal training in lasers. Dermatologists are trained to become experts of the skin and perform various procedures during residency but have little to no exposure to laser and cosmetic surgery. They have to apply and be accepted into fellowship programs for postgraduate training to specialize in laser and cosmetic surgery. There are very few programs that are accredited to provide training in laser and cosmetic surgery and they're very competitive. So one should not assume that a board-certified dermatologist has legitimate formal training in lasers. They may also have received their training from attending a weekend course. However, a board-certified dermatologist with no laser training would still be far preferable to a board-certified internist with no laser training. Even without adequate training in lasers, a dermatologist would at least know how to care for the skin in the event of complications such as burns and blisters resulting from the laser treatment.

A plastic surgeon is trained to perform reconstructive surgery, breast implantation and reduction surgery, rhinoplasties, abdomino-plasties (tummy-tucks) during residency training but do not receive exposure to laser procedures. The vast majority of plastic surgeons also would not have any training in lasers unless they went for further training in a fellowship program to specialize in lasers after residency. Most plastic surgeons also received their "training" from attending a weekend course. They would be less capable of diagnosing and caring for skin problems than a dermatologist if problems arose but much more capable than an internist or primary care physician.

There are many cases of patients who had melanoma which were mistakenly treated with laser by plastic surgeons and nurses, misdiagnosing the melanoma as a mole. This sort of mistake would not have occurred with a dermatologist.

I see a large number of complications from patients treated at dermatologist and plastic surgeon's offices. (This sadly is nothing compared to the complications seen arising from shadows and rogues though). These patients would ask in confusion, "How could this happen—I went to see a board-certified dermatologist (or plastic surgeon)." It's perplexing for the average consumer to understand how to select a proper laser surgeon when they often assume the key was to find a board-certified dermatologist or plastic surgeon. That is a very important factor but not the sole criteria. Many dermatologists and plastic surgeons have no formal training in lasers other than attending a weekend course and so they are "dabblers" when it comes to lasers. They buy or rent one or two lasers and don't have the full range of lasers that would be needed in order to provide the best and most comprehensive services. Their knowledge and repertoire is extremely limited. They may literally have just bought their laser after attending a weekend course and you may be the second or third patient they've ever treated. They're not clear about what types of complications can arise and how to avoid them. If a complication arises, they're not quite sure what to do (but they cause far less damage than an internist or OB/Gyn in the same situation).

A great example of a dabbler is a dermatologist who is well-known and established in the community for treating psoriasis but suddenly decides he wants to buy a laser and expand his repertoire. He advertises in all the papers that he has over 25 years of experience (this is a huge red flag in of itself because lasers haven't been around for 25 years). The ad is attempting to mislead the patient into believing that he has 25 years of experience performing lasers (not just doing general dermatology and treating psoriasis). He has an ad out for the "FotoFacial". The ad claims that the FotoFacial will remove sun damage, rosacea, freckles, blood vessels, acne scars, wrinkles, tighten the skin and make your pores disappear. During your consultation, you tell the doctor that your primary concern is wrinkles, large pores, and acne scarring. The doctor recommends a FotoFacial—he doesn't give you any other options. You then schedule another appointment and consultation with a true laser expert, a board-certified dermatologist who has fellowship training in lasers, extensive experience in performing laser procedures, and owns over 20 lasers. This doctor educates you on the various treatment options ranging from carbon dioxide (CO_2) laser, Erbium:YAG laser, dermabrasion, Thermage, Fraxel, and a multitude of noninvasive laser procedures that can be used in combination to achieve the best results. You ask yourself, why did the first doctor only talk about the FotoFacial? The answer is easy, because that doctor was a one trick pony—he only owned one laser so he would only push that one laser procedure no matter what your problem was. He is not able to educate you on the vast array of options you have and certainly is incapable of providing them.

Some easy questions to ascertain a physician's background and qualifications to perform laser procedures are as follows: (1) What is the doctor's board certification in? (2) Where did they get their training in lasers? Doesn't matter if the doctor is board-certified in internal medicine from Stanford and went to medical school at Harvard. Ask specifically where they got their training in lasers. Some doctors will try to skirt this question by saying they spent "some time" (could be one day or a week) with a "laser expert" at Harvard. Ask specifically if they did a fellowship in laser and cosmetic surgery. How long was this fellowship? Most fellowships are at least a year long. (3) How long have they been performing laser treatments? (4) How many people have they treated? (5) How many lasers do they own? (6) Ask to see before and after photos.

Complications can happen anywhere. Even in the hands of an expert, things can go wrong. But wouldn't you rather be in the best hands if something were to go wrong? During my fellowship, I was able to see the full gamut of what can go wrong and also got to see all the different complications that may occur in other people's hands. This gave me the confidence of knowing that I could deal with any incident or mishap if it were to occur. Someone who has not gone through a fellowship doesn't have proper appreciation or respect for all that can go wrong which is probably why they're so cavalier about performing procedures that they're not familiar with. If a doctor can't deal with the complications, they shouldn't be performing the procedure. A laser expert can avoid most of the complications by taking certain precautions that an untrained physician wouldn't know about. Complications are common occurrences in the hands of the inexperienced. And when they do occur, they don't even know what to do.

Patients can be their own worst enemy. I've had some patients who were noncompliant with instructions and caused harm to themselves after undergoing a laser procedure. Even in these situations, I was able to administer proper care to prevent permanent damage from occurring. In other words, I can help fix most things even if wrought by the patient's own carelessness. I know that a less experienced physician would not be able to do this.

Also, I possess the knowledge and skills to help patients who have suffered from complications resulting from poor or negligent care elsewhere by reversing the damage. I spend a great deal of time helping patients who have scarring or disfigurements caused by badly performed laser procedures done elsewhere. Many of these patients were lured in by lower prices and ads making unreal promises. I've had patients not sign up for procedures because they didn't like what they heard but I was telling them the truth. They would go shopping around until they finally had someone tell them what they wanted to hear even if it wasn't the truth. At best, they felt they were scammed and threw away their money. At worst, they were left maimed and scarred. And they would then have to pay even more to have someone else remove the damages, and that's if they were lucky enough to have damages that were reversible.

As I have already mentioned, I have formal training in lasers by completing an advanced fellowship program in addition to being a board-certified dermatologist. I have many years of experience, treated thousands of patients successfully with lasers, work with many of the top laser companies helping to develop and refine laser devices and procedures, lecture around the world, research and publish extensively, and teach at the University of California, San Francisco. I am a pioneer and researcher in laser and cosmetic surgery. I am also the pioneer and developer of several laser rejuvenation procedures. I also happen to own more than 25 lasers.

Common sense would dictate that as a recognized laser expert, I would have access to the best and widest range of lasers. I am constantly researching new lasers and am usually the first one to have access to them. If there is a new and better laser, I'm usually the first one to get it. I usually test the new lasers long before most other doctors even hear about them. As I go into greater detail in chapters 6 and 7, if I decided not to get a laser, there's usually a very good reason. Usually, the only reason I don't get a certain new brand of laser is because it doesn't do a better job than a preexisting laser. I recently heard of a couple of local family practitioners who practice together who were claiming that they had "the best" laser in the entire area. When the person asked them if they had heard of me, they said, "Oh, yeah, we've heard of her—she's good but we have 'the best' laser and she doesn't have that one." And amazing that they were claiming that their one laser was better than all the lasers I had. Because that supposes that their one laser would supplant the functions of more than 25 different lasers and in addition outperform each and every one of them.

As I mentioned in Chapter 3, Choosing a Doctor, a C+ doctor couldn't make an A+ laser perform to its highest potential. An A+ laser in the hands of a C+ doctor would give C+ results. So even if they actually had "the best" laser (and as you should realize from reading Chapter 2, Review of Lasers, there is no such thing as one best laser for everything), they couldn't possibly make it perform to its highest potential without the proper training.

A major warning sign that you are dealing with an amateur is a claim such as the one I mentioned above—that they try to sell you on the type of laser they have rather than on their training and experience and ability to use many different lasers in order to help optimize your results. A laser doesn't give you results—the qualified physician does. The laser is only as good as the practitioner operating it. You can have 10 different people utilizing a laser and get 10 different outcomes. Even if they were following a formula or recipe, there are so many individual nuances and variations between each individual that it's impossible to generalize about any laser procedure. A true laser master knows how to optimize each laser and combine various lasers in his or her armamentarium to suit the individual's needs.

Laser and cosmetic surgery is an art as well as a science. That's why it can never be mass produced or regulated to an assembly line. This is what laser spa/salon chains are attempting to do and they will always consistently fail at. People are investing vast amounts of money in this industry thinking they can cash in on the cosmetic boom but these businesses inevitably fail due to complications and inability to provide long-term customer satisfaction.

One may ask that if these businesses will inevitably fail, why not let the market control itself? Why bother to close them down? I used to think that way back in 2000 and 2001 when I observed the first few chains come and go. One of the largest ones was **Vanishing Point** in San Francisco. They used to run full page ads in the San Francisco newspapers advertising laser hair removal at ridiculously low prices. They were funded by ESC, which supplied all their IPL devices. They did well initially because they were able to sign up a lot of customers for bargain basement prepaid package deals. But once they had to start doing the treatments, they soon realized they couldn't afford to pay their expenses after charging such low prices. They closed down after a year and left their customers with unfulfilled package agreements that were already paid for. They declared bankruptcy to escape from the impending lawsuits.

I thought that would be the end of it because surely the public and investors would see what a poor business model these laser salons were and stay away. Boy, was I wrong. They have just kept proliferating and despite each chain following the same fate as Vanishing Point, there are always 3 more to take the place of the one that goes out of business. It's amazing that people never learn. Hope runs eternal with people foolishly throwing their money away at these things. The public and investors all lose out. The only true benefactor from these boondoggles has been the laser companies. They love it when chains buy their lasers and then go out of business. They don't have to maintain the service contracts on lasers whose owners have gone out of business. The more turnover there is in the business, the more lasers they'll sell. They may only sell one laser to one doctor in a 10 year period if that doctor stays in business for 10 years. But if a salon closes down annually and is replaced with another salon, they'll sell a new laser every year when there's a new salon that opens. That could be 10 laser sales in a 10 year period if there's a new salon opening for every salon that closes each year. Multiply that by the exponential increase of laser sales to nonphysicians.

Every new chain thinks that they have the magic formula for success where the previous laser salon chain failed. The reason they can never succeed is because laser treatments are medical treatments that cannot be mass produced like McDonald's. There can be no "McLaser". Laser treatments have to be individualized to each patient. No two patients can be treated alike. No two people have the identical skin conditions or problems (unless they are identical twins—even then, there may be exceptions. For example, one of the twins may have a skin cancer).

I would recommend that investors stay away from laser salon and medspa franchising opportunities. These are poor business strategies doomed to fail and worse than losing your investment dollars, when the business shuts down, there's a blaze of victims left in their wake. Few other failing businesses cause their victims to be both financially and physically damaged.

About 90% of the practitioners performing laser procedures are shadows, rogues, or dabblers. That may be shocking to the consumer but there's a logical reason why. The laser companies need to sell lasers in order to survive. If they only catered to doctors properly trained to perform lasers that would be an incredibly small pool indeed. They would probably go out of business. Even if they sold only to dermatologists that probably still wouldn't be enough to sustain their business. The market of untrained practitioners is a much bigger one so the laser companies go after them. They are part of the problem—they try to convince non-cosmetically trained physicians to purchase a laser by saying they'll help train them (by sending them to a weekend course) and tantalizing them with the promise of additional cash revenue the laser will bring into their practice. Laser companies weren't even content with peddling their wares to nontrained physicians —they have continually tried expanding their market to include nonphysicians, salons and spas.

An enterprising lawyer could easily file a class action lawsuit against the laser companies who sell lasers to nonphysicians, salons and spas. These laser companies are violating Food and Drug Administration (FDA) regulations which classify lasers as medical prescription devices which can only be sold to physicians. Laser companies are the ultimate culprits involved in aiding and abetting the nonphysician practice of medicine. They market their lasers to unqualified and untrained physicians and nurses who fool themselves into believing they can receive adequate training in a day seminar or course. They sell them the laser with some marketing materials and instruction manuals, and before you know it, they're advertising in the local paper. Their patients are literally guinea pigs for these novices to practice their newly acquired toys on. Do you want to be some numbskull's first laser victim? If the answer is no, then make sure you read this book thoroughly!

Chapter 6:

Cutting thru the Hype of Marketing, Ads, and the Media

VISIA BY CANFIELD IS an imaging system that uses an ultraviolet (UV) light to highlight sun damage in computerized digital images. A local dermatologist appeared on the local news showing the VISIA system in his practice. He was using it to demonstrate the effectiveness of the IPL or "FotoFacial" for removing sun damage. It was obvious to me that the before and after photos he used were misleading because it showed very severe sun damage in the before picture, the after picture showed complete removal of all sun damage. A lay person would be easily deceived by this. The IPL is not used directly over the eyelids so it would have been impossible for the sun damage to somehow disappear in the after photo. The only thing that would account for this discrepancy would be that the patient had make-up on in the after photo and had no make-up in the before photo.

No make-up in the before photo and wearing make-up or foundation in the after photo is an old gimmick which can readily be detected in normal photography. It's impossible for the layperson to see whether there is make-up being used in the VISIA imaging system because the computerized digital images appear through a UV filter, which highlights only sun damage. You can mimic the effects of the UV filter by standing in the dark and shining a blue fluorescent bulb over your face—it makes you look like you have a fluorescent glow with lots of white specks highlighting the areas of greatest sun damage on your face. If you have make-up on and shine the light, it appears as if your sun damage has magically disappeared. The VISIA system can be easily manipulated to fool patients into thinking they have remarkable results which in reality may be nonexistent. The bottom line is: if you can't see the results easily just by viewing standard or digital before and after photos, then it doesn't really matter what a computerized program shows you. Doctors who have to rely on these sophisticated diagnostic tools often do so only because they can't clearly demonstrate through standard photos that there was a significant improvement so they have to embellish by adding bells and whistles to distract from the lack of real results.

The proper usage of the VISIA system or any other photography system would require complete removal of make-up prior to any photo being taken. Have you ever noticed on ABC's Extreme Makeover that the before and after photos are always done with the person looking their worst without any benefit of make-up or hairstyling in the before photo, and then they have elaborate make-up and hairstyling in the after photo? Forget about all the plastic surgery, the make-up and hair and flattering clothes make the greatest difference.

Before and after photos are crucial, however, because many people forget what they looked like before they started the laser treatments. Many laser treatments require a series of multiple treatments and the results occur slowly over a period of time, so it's easy for the patient to lose track of the transformation that is occurring. If you're looking at yourself everyday in the mirror, you're less apt to notice significant changes than someone else who hasn't seen you for a few months who can easily detect that you've gone through a dramatic improvement. Many patients report that friends, family, colleagues tell them they can see a huge improvement if they haven't seen them for awhile after they finished a series of laser treatments. It's amazing how people develop a sort of amnesia when it comes to remembering how bad they looked to begin with. No one seems to want to admit that they had wrinkles and splotches. When I show patients their before and after photos, they're often shocked at the memory of how bad their skin looked in the before photos and say, "Yuck! Throw that picture away! I never want to see it again!" They're in total denial that they ever looked that bad which is odd, because it begs to ask, if your skin was perfect to begin with, why did you elect to go through these treatments?

Nevertheless, patients are thrilled to see the before and after photos because it helps them to clearly visualize the improvements that have taken place. It's also important from the standpoint of documenting that certain imperfections may have been existent before undergoing treatments. For example, some patients may never have noticed they had a particular scar on their face prior to treatment. After starting laser treatments, they start scrutinizing their face more and suddenly notice that they have a scar and may attribute that to a complication from the laser treatment. Having the before photo helps to reassure the patient that the scar was indeed present before the treatments and was not created by the laser.

One of my patients looked 20 years younger after going through carbon dioxide (CO2) laser resurfacing. She was 50 years old at the time she underwent CO2 resurfacing and looked like Paul McCartney (an older Paul McCartney). After undergoing laser, she looked better than she did in her 30's because she had never had good skin even when she was young due to acne scarring. She said the most disturbing thing to her was noticing how people, especially men, treated her so differently. She had young grocery clerks running to help assist her with carrying groceries to her car where she had never had anyone offer before. It actually made her mad and want to say to them, "What's the deal? They used to always ignore me when I was old and ugly...so I wanted to give them a piece of my mind!" And her teenage sons' classmates voted her the "hottest babe Mom" of all the mothers in their class. What a huge compliment!

Her husband's reaction exemplifies the difficult position that men are in that they can never say anything right when it comes to a woman's appearance. She said that if her husband had tried ignoring the fact that she underwent a drastic procedure and didn't comment on her new appearance, she would have been devastated that he didn't notice. But since her husband told her she looked great and beautiful, she yelled at him, "So what was wrong with the way I looked before?"

Some of the most egregious manipulation of before and after photos were used in promoting nonablative resurfacing procedures such as the NLite and CoolTouch procedures which came out around 1999 and 2000. These nonablative procedures were touted as being the "Holy Grail" to replace CO_2 ablative resurfacing for removing wrinkles. There were some claims that the results surpassed those of the CO_2 laser without any downtime. Sounds too good to be true? It was.

The photos used to advertise the NLite and CoolTouch showed close-ups only of the crow's feet which were so closely cropped that you couldn't tell that the before photo was of the patient smiling and the after photo was of the patient relaxed. So you can imagine how dramatic that would appear. Smoke and mirrors. Good reliable photos should always show the before and after photo of the same person (yes, believe it or not, some companies have used before and after photos of different people!), full-face, no make-up, same angle and profile and view, same lighting, and same facial expression.

Another popular advertising gimmick is using normal direct lighting in the before photo to highlight wrinkles and defects, while the after photo is using overexposed lighting which makes the photo appear washed out so it appears as if all the wrinkles and defects have disappeared. I have demonstrated this in lectures where I showed before and after photos of people who had no treatments performed but looked 20 years younger just by varying lighting and facial expression and angles.

A couple of physicians doing seminars for a laser company had an advertising brochure for their procedure depicting a before photo of a 60-ish woman in a split-face comparison with an obviously 20-ish woman which was supposed to be the after result, claiming that the improvements were achieved with their laser procedure.

Other companies and physicians have obviously altered or "Photoshopped" their after photos. A trained eye can usually spot the telltale signs. Disappearance of moles or other distinguishing landmarks, areas of improvement that couldn't be treated with the laser (i.e., in the case of the Fraxel laser—there was a before and after photo which showed obvious digital alteration of the eye area which was obvious because the Fraxel couldn't be used directly over the eye area). Also, as in the case of the VISIA system example above, one should be very suspicious of a patient reportedly getting IPL or "FotoFacial" who showed disappearance of brown spots and blood vessels over the eyelids because the IPL can't be used to treat directly over the eyelids.

Every other week there seems to be the discovery of the new "Holy Grail." This term has been so overused that it's become meaningless. Every nonablative laser has been described as the Holy Grail and last year it was used to describe the Fraxel laser. It was described in Allure magazine as the Holy Grail of lasers—they said it produced results better than the CO2 laser with no downtime. Sound familiar? Once again, if it sounds too good to be true, it probably is.

The IPL or "FotoFacial" was also described as the Holy Grail when it first came out. The manufacturers claimed the device did everything from removing sun damage, rosacea, broken blood vessels, pigmentation, wrinkles, acne scars, diminished pores, and tightened the skin. It does provide significant reduction of sun damage, rosacea, and pigmentation, but it barely has any effect on wrinkles or pore size or tightening of the skin.

The evolution of the IPL device has been fascinating. It first came out as the Photoderm (nicknamed the "Photoburn" because there were so many complications) and it never really caught on. It was reborn in the late 90's with an aggressive marketing strategy by Lumenis. The doctor who popularized the "FotoFacial" learned how to perform the procedure from another doctor by going for a preceptorship. He came up with a catchy name and hence the "FotoFacial" was born. That doctor went on to conduct countless seminars and workshops, and "trained" countless doctors, nurses, and "interested parties". This doctor was very nondiscriminating in who attended his seminars and was probably most responsible for starting the trend of promoting lasers (or light devices) to non-cosmetically trained doctors and nonphysicians.

I have developed a laser procedure as well which involves the combination of two different wavelengths: the KTP 532 nm and Nd:YAG 1064 nm lasers.[1,2] I was asked by the laser company who manufacturers these lasers to give lectures and seminars to doctors introducing the new procedure. At the beginning, I wasn't aware of how many nondermatologists would be attending these seminars. After becoming aware of the encroachment of nonspecialists and nonphysicians who tried to acquire minimal "laser training" by attending these lectures, I then limited my lectures and seminars to only dermatologists and plastic surgeons and other cosmetically trained specialists. I use the word "laser training" loosely because attending an 8 hour lecture or seminar does not constitute legitimate laser training. It's like taking a page from Cliff Notes and saying it's as good as reading the entire book.

I only allow dermatologists and plastic surgeons in my office for preceptorships. These are instructional sessions for doctors who come from all over the U.S. and other countries who want to observe an expert at work and treatment techniques. These doctors are allowed to visit my practice and observe me treating patients. The doctor leaves with some basic understanding of the laser procedures performed that day with tips for settings and treatment protocols, pre- and post-procedural care. A dermatologist can get a lot more out of a preceptorship than a noncosmetically trained physician.

I knew from my early exposure to IPL devices that their effects were much more limited than certain lasers. Its ability to clear pigmented lesions and blood vessels is inferior to that of the KTP 532 nm green wavelength laser. The KTP laser is more specific for brown and red pigment and penetrates into the skin much deeper therefore providing better clearance of lesions. The KTP laser is the gold standard for removing vascular and pigmented lesions. There were several KTP lasers on the market in 1998 when I was in my fellowship training. Laserscope, Iriderm, and Lumenis (originally Coherent) all had KTP lasers. Lumenis was the merger of ESC/Sharplan with Coherent, which resulted in the world's largest laser company at that time. ESC was known for developing the IPL device (the original Photoderm). Lumenis had also acquired Coherent's Versapulse in the merger. The Versapulse was a great laser comprised of 4 different lasers: variable pulsed KTP laser (for vascular and pigmented lesions), Q-switched KTP (for red tattoos), Q-switched Nd:YAG (for black tattoos), and Q-switched Alexandrite (for black, blue, and green tattoos). This was an extremely versatile laser but was very costly to manufacture and broke down a lot due to the sensitive computerized screen. The profit margin to Lumenis was much lower with the Versapulse compared to the IPL. The Versapulse cost about $50,000 to produce and sold for about $150,000. The IPL Quantum cost about $10,000 to produce and sold for about $150,000. So you can see that the profit margin was so much higher that Lumenis didn't have much incentive to continue manufacturing and promoting the Versapulse. They would much rather sell a lot more IPL devices. So they launched an aggressive marketing campaign to promote the IPL device which cannibalized their other products including the Versapulse. The Versapulse is an intricate series of lenses and fiberoptics and laser optics. Lasers involve expensive crystals and lenses and intricate fiberoptics. The IPL handpiece is an inexpensive glass prism or filter—it's not a laser at all. It's really a light device. Lasers are much more expensive to make, break down a lot, and require constant maintenance. IPL's on the other hand are really low tech, inexpensive to make, rarely break down, and require little maintenance.

Lumenis dominated the market for a couple years while there was a "FotoFacial" craze. Everyone was jumping on the bandwagon. There were wild unsubstantiated claims being made about the "FotoFacial". I knew that the laser procedure I developed was far more effective than the IPL procedure, but understood that hype and advertising were driving the market. I spent most of my time trying to educate patients about the difference between photorejuvenation using IPL vs. lasers. I knew that over time, patients and physicians would come to realize the limitations of IPL treatments. I have countless patients who have gone for countless IPL treatments and have hit the ceiling in terms of being able to achieve any further results. At this point, they need laser treatments in order to progress further. I have one patient who had more than 20 IPL treatments performed by the developer of the "FotoFacial". She was unhappy with the treatment results and came to me for the dual laser procedure that I had developed for photorejuvenation. She said she got better results from 2 laser procedures in my practice than she had from over 20 FotoFacials. She went on to finish a series of 6 laser procedures and achieved clearance in her rosacea that she would never have been able to achieve with FotoFacials no matter how many treatments were performed.

The bottom dropped out of Lumenis' market when other companies started developing IPL devices and offering them at far lower prices than Lumenis. Lumenis' stock dropped from a high of $40+ down to less than $1 and became delisted from the New York Stock Exchange.

Even the doctor who originally coined the "FotoFacial" name jumped ship from Lumenis and teamed up with Syneron to promote the "FotoFacial Plus". The Syneron devices were a combination of IPL with bipolar radiofrequency. The claim was that the radiofrequency energy helped make the IPL more effective and safer, and therefore the treatment results were superior to the original IPL. I found in practice that the results are better for hair removal and clearance of pigmentation, rosacea, and sun damage, but that it still didn't have appreciable effects on wrinkles or skin tightening. It also did not perform as well as the KTP laser. The major limitation of the Syneron IPL/RF device was the same as with any IPL device—that the handpiece is too large and awkward for treating curvaceous areas around the face especially the nose, which is where the predominance of large blood vessels and pigmentation need to be treated. And since the IPL is not a focused beam like the laser, it's far less effective on individual blood vessels and pigmented lesions. Liken the IPL to blasting the entire forest but not capable of targeting specific trees. Many people have small discrete lesions (i.e., individual blood vessels or moles or freckles) that they would like removed—it's not possible to remove a 2 mm round lesion with a 1 x 1 cm handpiece without causing a white imprint around that small lesion. Also, the filter is like a big block that needs to be held over the lesion so you can't visualize the lesion while it's being treated. It's like performing surgery with a sledgehammer.

With the advent of cheap IPL devices, the "FotoFacial" boom started in Asia. Taiwan and Hong Kong bought up IPL devices, favoring them over lasers, due mostly to cost, not to the effectiveness of the devices. They paid little attention to laser physics and studies which would guide a physician to intuitively understand that lasers are more effective than IPL. They cared more about the bottom line and preferred to buy the cheaper devices. Over the years, they have finally come to discover that the IPL devices are limited in the results that can be achieved and people are looking for more. So now they are turning towards lasers. They are just now starting to buy and perform more laser procedures. They tend to lag behind the U.S. by about 5 years in terms of laser technology and usage.

After the IPL and nonablative craze, next came the Thermage phenomenon. This device is a radiofrequency device, not a laser or a light. It utilizes the same electrical energy that is used in electrocautery devices which have been used for more than a hundred years while performing surgery to stop bleeding. Electrocautery devices deliver monopolar or bipolar electric radiowaves which thermocoagulate (burn) blood vessels causing a clot to form and seal the blood vessels in order to stop blood flow. Thermage is a company devoted solely to manufacturing one device, the ThermaCool. This is a monopolar radiofrequency device, meaning that the electrical energy is delivered in one direction and the patient is grounded in order for the electrical energy to pass through the patient.

Bipolar radiofrequency is used in the Syneron devices, not to be confused with monopolar radiofrequency used in the Thermage devices. They are completely different. Bipolar radiofrequency involves two metal prongs that deliver a closed circuit wave of electrical energy. The energy passes from one metal prong and is returned in a circular arc back through the other prong after passing through the skin. The patient does not need to be grounded when using bipolar radiofrequency. However, if the two prongs are not in contact with the patient's skin surface, the electrical impulse can arc above the skin causing a shock resulting in burn to the skin.

The Thermage device was released in 2002 with a huge wave of excitement and hype. Proponents of the procedure claimed it was like a nonsurgical facelift and could possibly put plastic surgeons out of business. And yes, you guessed it, they claimed it was the elusive Holy Grail. We all marveled at the notion of tightening the skin without any downtime. In reality, this procedure does cause tightening of the skin, but not as much as people hoped. The device does work, just not to the degree that it was hyped up to do. The problem with any procedure or device has been in establishing realistic expectations. Who wouldn't want the exact same results as a facelift without undergoing the knife. That's a no-brainer. But what if the doctor told you that you'd have to pay several thousand dollars and only get about 30% tightening?

I have found from my practice that the average patient gets around 30% tightening with the Thermage procedure. In my estimation, that's pretty darn good. Just not good enough for those who have already been tainted by the marketing hype. After the media and advertisers have preprogrammed the consumer to expect miracles, the doctor (who's honest) has the unfortunate job of educating the patient about the realities of a procedure, and they're never as good as they sound in the magazines.

Which brings us to the next point—the role the media plays in educating patients (or mis-educating might be more accurate). Reporters constantly interview physicians and industry officials, trying to get the next big story. They want every story to be the "Holy Grail". That's what sells newspapers and magazines. Reporters tend to over hype the good things and underplay the bad in their attempt to generate excitement about a new product or procedure. Not many people would buy a magazine that said, "Read about the new ho-hum device that gives so-so results". But most new lasers are exactly that. Very few earth-shattering inventions are ever made—they come around very infrequently and you can bet that when they do, the results are startling and they don't require hype to sell because the results speak for themselves.

The CO_2 laser was a home run. Its results were irrefutable and obvious. You didn't need a VISIA or in-vivo imaging system to convince yourself that there were changes in the before and after photos. The results obtained with CO_2 laser were dramatic and the patients receiving this procedure easily looked 20 years younger. But it's an invasive laser which involves considerable downtime and increased risks, especially if not performed by a qualified physician.

In terms of results, the CO_2 laser is a home run for removing wrinkles. It has the major drawback of being invasive and requiring considerable downtime, so it's not the Holy Grail that we're all seeking. The KTP laser is a home run for treating vascular (blood vessels) and pigmented (brown) lesions. After that, I can't think of any other home runs. Everything else is either a first, second, or third base hit. The thinking with the nonablative lasers (i.e., NLite, CoolTouch, SmoothBeam, etc.) was that they were base hits but if you hit enough base hits, you'll eventually get home. Not true. You could do a hundred

NLite treatments and it still won't come close to the results of one CO2 laser procedure.

After the CO2 phenomenon, the next major development was the Erbium:YAG 2940 nm laser. Like the CO2 laser, it targets water in the skin and causes vaporization (or removal) of the top layer of skin. The Erbium laser does not go as deep as the CO2 laser, therefore its healing time is decreased, but so are the results. The Erbium laser is a good alternative to the CO2 laser for patients who are younger, have less deep wrinkles, and also for darker ethnic patients who may have greater risk of complications with the CO2 laser. It's also ideal for resurfacing more sensitive areas such as the neck, chest, and hands.

One of the biggest slights of hand that occurred within the laser industry was the development of the nonablative lasers and the hype associated with them. Several years ago, a dermatologist and noted laser expert published a paper about an observation she made that when treating vascular lesions with the pulsed dye laser, that she noted improvements in wrinkles.[3] Years later, the NLite came onto the scene. It is a pulsed dye laser (yellow wavelength) that is typically used to treat blood vessels. It got repackaged in a new box and labeled as a "new" device to remove wrinkles in a noninvasive manner. It was touted to be the "Holy Grail" and isn't it amazing that the Holy Grail was right under our nose the whole time? The series of events that followed were quite amusing (if not confounding) for laser industry insiders to follow—it became clear that the Emperor had no clothes.

The NLite was an old laser repackaged to sound like a new laser with new applications. Dermatologists then got wise to the idea and decided to turn all their other pulsed dye lasers into anti-aging nonablative lasers. The physiologic basis for nonablative resurfacing was that the pulsed dye laser stimulated collagen production by heating the dermis. All of a sudden, the "old" lasers became the newest technological phenomena. Candela is the major manufacturer of pulsed dye lasers. They decided to jump on the bandwagon by relabeling all of their pulsed dye lasers as nonablative lasers. The Vbeam and Cbeam are both pulsed dye lasers traditionally known as vascular lasers which magically became nonablative overnight.

The CoolTouch then came along soon after the NLite and also claimed the right to be one of the first nonablative lasers to remove wrinkles with no downtime. The CoolTouch is a 1320 nm Nd:YAG (infrared) laser that stimulates collagen remodeling by heating the dermis (just like the NLite). The company would show histologic photos (highly magnified images of the skin taken under a microscope) which showed layers of new collagen being formed after being treated with the laser. These photos were exactly like the photos shown by the company which made the NLite. Both companies showed closely cropped photos of the crow's feet showing them completely gone afterward. (It was obvious to the trained eye that these photos were of patients smiling and not smiling in many cases). In many cases there were genuine improvements but they were usually for very fine wrinkles and also they were not sustained. Most patients required multiple treatments to get the best results, the results would usually last only a few months, and then they required continual maintenance treatments.

It then became obvious that any laser, regardless of wavelength, should be capable of inducing the same changes. There's nothing specific about the pulsed dye laser or the Nd:YAG laser that would allow them exclusive rights to claim that only their laser was able to stimulate collagen production. It turns out that every laser is capable of stimulating collagen production and therefore improving wrinkles. The question then is how much wrinkle reduction? In reality, the results have not been able to compete with the results achieved with the CO_2 or Erbium:YAG resurfacing lasers.

After the advent of the NLite and CoolTouch, all the other laser companies jumped on the bandwagon to take advantage of the nonablative craze and repackaged and relabeled their preexisting lasers as "nonablative". What the consumer needs to know is that there isn't just one nonablative laser that is head and shoulders above the rest. They're all basically the same. The principles are all based upon collagen stimulation and production of new collagen and elastic fibers which can "plump" up the skin and make the wrinkles look better. They also help with acne scarring.

Every laser company has a nonablative laser. Many of these lasers have multiple applications such as hair removal, leg veins, vascular and pigmented lesions. Old lasers were revamped to sound like the new kid on the block. It seemed like every week there was a "new" laser being released which wasn't a new laser, just a new application or repackaging of a preexisting laser.

The next progression in laser evolution was the discovery that all lasers also help treat acne. It had been noted anecdotally by many practitioners that all their lasers seemed to incidentally help acne while they were treating other conditions such as performing laser hair removal or photorejuvenation. The first light device that received FDA approval for acne treatment was the ClearLight by Lumenis. First is not always the best—it turned out that this device was far less effective than the laser that received FDA approval later. The first laser to receive FDA approval was the SmoothBeam by Candela. The SmoothBeam is a 1450 nm (infrared) diode laser which is absorbed predominately by water. It was originally promoted as a nonablative laser but then turned out to be effective for treating acne.

All the other nonablative lasers eventually received FDA approval for treating acne. Hair removal lasers received FDA clearance for being nonablative. Nonablative lasers received FDA clearance for treating acne. Hair removal lasers received FDA clearance for treating acne. Light devices received FDA clearance for nonablative, acne, and hair removal.

Many of the principles which make a hair removal device good at targeting hair, also makes that device good for targeting collagen and stimulating collagen production, and also makes it effective for treating acne. But there is great variability between the lasers that make some better for treating some conditions more than others (see Chapter 2: Review of Lasers). Not all lasers are created equally and it's certainly true that some are the Jack-of-All-Trades but the Master-of-None.

Then came the Thermage phenomenon—lead by the need for a device that tightened the skin. The nonablative lasers provided modest wrinkle reduction but minimal to no tightening of the skin. There was a perceived gap in the nonablative armamentarium that the Thermage device seemed to fill.

Having used the Thermage device for over 4 years, I have found that there is great variability with the results. The early studies showed that there was a 20% nonresponder rate. This means that out of 100 patients, 20 patients would have no response. This nonresponder rate was eliminated by performing more treatments and performing more passes (the number of times you go over the face) on each treatment. The problem with this treatment was that many doctors were trying to sign up more patients by overselling the results or by lowering the price (which would necessitate skimping on the treatment, doing less passes) and not recommending multiple treatments in order to make the procedure appear more affordable. The patient should understand that to perform this procedure to its optimal level, it would take at least 1-1/2 to 2-1/2 hours to go over the entire face 6 to 9 times. The longer the procedure takes, the more it will cost. If you cut corners by trying to get a minimal treatment, the results will reflect that. A reasonable price to charge for this procedure would be $2500-$4500, especially if it's performed by the doctor. It someone's charging less than that and taking less time, you can be certain that the procedure is not being performed to its optimal level.

In my practice, I undersell the procedure and I over deliver. I take the Scotty (from Star Trek) approach with Captain Kirk. Whenever Captain Kirk asked Scotty how long it would take for him to fix the Enterprise, Scotty would say something like, "I can't do it before 24 hours, Captain." And Captain Kirk would say, "You've only got 12, Scotty." And somehow Scotty would come through because he knew better than to tell the Captain that he actually could do it in 8. He undersold and over delivered.

I'm very candid with patients about the results. I tell them that if they don't see any results after the first Thermage treatment, then they need to do a second treatment. I've not had a single patient not have a response after doing at least 2 treatments. Many patients truly can't tell how much improvement they've had until you show them their before and after photos because so much time has elapsed between treatments and they tend to forget what they looked like. The most important thing is making sure you don't have unrealistically high expectations to begin with.

There is such great variability in Thermage results. The better re-sponding patients are those with thinner skin with mobility. A good test is seeing if the skin moves easily over the forehead bone. If the skin is fixed and doesn't move, then you're less likely to get a noticeable browlift from the procedure. Same with the cheeks and jawline. If you can easily move the skin over the underlying bone, then you're a good candidate.

There have been some patients with truly amazing results with the Thermage. They look like a home run. If every patient looked like these patients, this procedure truly would be the Holy Grail. Unfortunately, these "miracle" patients comprise a very small subset of the whole. After performing the Thermage procedure for more than 4 years, I have found that the average treatment result is around 30% but the range is 10-70%. This means that some patients have as low as 10% improvement but others have as high as 70% improvement.

Companies tend to show their best photos and report the higher range of the results. For example, their research may show that a laser produces 10-90% improvement, with the average being around 30%. When you look at the actual data, you see that out of 100 patients, the bell-shaped curved fell around 30% but that there was one outlier that went up to 90%. Statisticians might even call this an anomaly and throw that number out. But then their marketing department will spin the results to highlight that the laser will provide "up to 90% improvement". The media will pick up on that press release and all the magazines will run articles about how this new amazing laser has produced up to 90% clearance of wrinkles "according to scientific research". And the company will display the one photo out of 100 that shows astounding results. If you had reviewed all 100 photos, you would see that most patients had so-so results and that one person was an anomaly.

This sort of marketing hype that is released by the company and furthered by the media is creating unrealistic expectations in the general public and setting patients up for disappointment. It's frustrating for an honest and ethical physician to have to counter what patients are reading in magazines. When I tell people the truth, they truly look disappointed. And the problem is that the lasers do actually work but they can never live up to the hype that has been created around them. I do not have a single laser that does not perform up to my expectations of what it should do based on the actual scientific research. But the truth is far from what people want to hear.

The problem is that if someone shops around enough, they'll eventually find someone who tells them what they want to hear, even if it's not true. There are a large number of doctors who do business by overselling their procedures in order to get people to sign up for them. I have talked to patients who claimed that they had no results from having the Thermage procedure done elsewhere. Upon questioning, I found out that they were told they would only have to do one procedure and that they only did one or 2 passes over their face and the price they were charged reflected that. They admitted that they chose that doctor because of the lower price. But then they were disappointed that they had no results.

What I find very sad is that I continually get patients coming back to tell me that they had to learn the hard way. They told me that they didn't like what I told them and they called around until they found a doctor that told them something that sounded more like what they wanted to hear. They went to that doctor only to find that in the end, the results were what I had described. And then they realized that I had been honest with them. I hear this continually with laser hair removal. Some laser clinics misrepresent themselves by advertising that their laser is better than all other lasers because they "guarantee" that all your hairs will be gone after only one treatment. This confuses the consumer who wonders why other doctors are telling them that laser hair removal is an ongoing process which requires multiple treatments and that the hairs will never be 100% gone. They mistakenly think that somehow these other laser clinics have a better laser and have discovered a treatment that's far superior to these other doctors saying you need multiple treatments. They soon find out that they've been lied to. Those clinics run on the philosophy that there's a sucker born every minute so they don't care if you feel burned and never come back. They don't have a business based on repeat customers. They're counting on having a high volume of new customers attracted to their low prices and ridiculous claims. So if it sounds too good to be true, it is!

I've actually lost customers because I refused to lie to them and would not give in to their demands to offer guarantees that I knew that I could not deliver. I would rather have a customer leave because they didn't like hearing the truth, rather than trying to butter them up, collect their money, and have them leave disappointed later. Remember, con men make a living by giving people what they want to hear.

The sad part of being those who have been conned is that they start to not believe in the technology, instead of thinking that they weren't given the proper information. I see many patients who have not been properly educated that blood vessels may require multiple treatments to clear. After they had one treatment and the blood vessels around their nose didn't clear up, they simply assumed that the laser didn't work. Even if the proper laser was used, the patient should have been told that they would need multiple treatments. If the blood vessels didn't clear after multiple treatments, then either the wrong laser or settings were used.

Too often, people blame treatment failures on the laser rather than on the practitioner either misinforming them or mistreating them. It's the practitioner's responsibility to be able to properly educate the patient on what the realistic expectations are from any procedure, and possible risks or complications.

An uninformed physician who's not knowledgeable or trained in lasers might easily be conned by a laser company representative who's willing to say anything to sell the laser. The laser rep might over hype the laser's capabilities which the doctor will in turn repeat to his patients. The doctor slowly discovers that he's been sold a bill of goods that he can't deliver. His patients start complaining that the laser's not working and the doctor is at a loss as to explain why because he really doesn't understand what the laser is truly capable of, nor has he properly researched the laser or how to use it.

I started seeing patients who were complaining that a local plastic surgeon's office was telling them that all their brown spots would be removed with only one treatment with their laser. The plastic surgeon had his nurse performing the procedures. I happened to know that the plastic surgeon had just purchased his first laser and neither he nor his nurse had any formal training or experience with lasers. His nurse was telling everyone that the brown spots would be "guaranteed" to be gone after only one treatment. (Amazing since no other laser or doctor has been able to perform this miracle!) She was probably just repeating what the laser rep had told them. It's possible that this could occur in 1 in 100 cases (that most likely being a very superficial freckle—the deeper the lesion is, the more treatments will be required to adequately remove it. And people have pigmented lesions of all different sizes and depth so there's no way to make generalized claims about being able to clear "all lesions" such as she did.) One patient in particular relayed to me that after the brown spot wasn't improved at all after one treatment, she went back and the nurse seemed perplexed and said, "I guess it just doesn't work on your skin type." She then performed a second treatment. Still no change. So the patient went back for a third treatment. Still no change. Back for a fourth treatment. The nurse turned up the setting and caused a blister and burn which left a scar.

I knew the exact laser that they were using—it wasn't a laser at all, it was an IPL device. It also left a white imprint around the lesion because the handpiece was a rectangle that was much bigger than the brown spot. It was definitely not the proper device to be treating her specific problem. And the only reason she chose to go to them was because they were the only ones claiming that they could remove the brown spot with only one treatment.

I have spoken with many doctors who complained to me that their laser rep had sold them their hair removal laser claiming that it would also treat leg veins. These doctors were easily conned because they didn't understand basic laser principles. If they did, they would have known that the particular wavelengths of their lasers were not conducive to treating leg veins. Their poor patients really suffered because after experimenting on their patients, they found out the hard way that their hair removal laser did absolutely nothing for leg veins.

The most recent claim being made by a laser company about its hair removal device really made me realize that we have come full circle from the nonablative craze. Candela has a long-pulsed 1064 nm Nd: YAG (infrared) laser called the GentleYAG which is used for hair removal on dark skin. We have already established that any laser can be used for nonablative resurfacing or collagen production. Candela has now repackaged their GentleYAG laser as the newest thing in skin tightening. In fact, they have a doctor claiming that it does better skin tightening than the Thermage procedure. From a scientific standpoint, this doesn't make any sense because it was established early on that none of the nonablative lasers did significant skin tightening. But it's almost as if they're counting on everyone having such short memories that we'll forget that we've already been down this path before. This would be like the NLite or CoolTouch repackaging itself now as a skin tightening procedure. (Which I really wouldn't be surprised if that happened).

Similar to the events occurring with the nonablative craze, every laser company is trying to come up with their version of the Thermage skin tightening procedure. But from a physics standpoint, it makes sense that the Thermage device causes skin tightening because it penetrates so deeply. And the theory behind tissue tightening has been that there needs to be deeper and more uniform heating than what nonablative lasers have been offering. Which explains why nonablative lasers were not effective for skin tightening. So it's almost comical to suddenly turn around and claim that these same nonablative lasers woke up one day and magically turned into skin tightening devices. The spin doctors are hard at work again.

Like any other company, Thermage may have over promoted the effects of its device. Some patients will get dramatic tightening but most patients will get around 30% tightening, but that's still significant. It's impossible to predict how any individual will respond because there's such great variability. You'll always hear about that one person who looked dramatically better after only one treatment but they're definitely the exception. Feel fortunate if that happens to you but don't expect it. The best results are achieved when the Thermage procedure is combined with other procedures (see Chapter 8).

Laser companies and their marketing departments will pour through thousands of cases to find the best results to highlight as being "typical" of their laser procedure. If they showed only their average pictures, they would never sell any lasers and doctors would never be able to get patients to sign up for procedures. I would be able to sign up every patient if I showed only the best results. Instead, I take great strides to show patients a great range of photos—I display the best, average, and worst responders so they can fully appreciate the full range of variability. I think a good sign that a doctor is being honest and ethical is if they're only signing up half of their patients. The initial consultation and education of patients is a weeding-out process--to filter through those patients who aren't good candidates or don't have realistic expectations. If the doctor is doing this well, they shouldn't be signing everyone up. They should be turning off a reasonable number of patients.

I spend hours upon hours on a regular basis with various reporters to help them write articles for media outlets such as magazines and newspapers. I provide them with accurate and informative material that would be indispensable for educating the public. My goal is to help reporters write articles that will be accurate and effective at educating the readers. Despite all my efforts, I am constantly dismayed at the hack jobs that they turn into. Often this is not the fault of the reporter but of the editor. They turn into puff pieces that are contrite and barely resemble the original material. Everything of substance has been edited out that would have helped you decide not to do a treatment or buy a product. The magazines seem more concerned to excite readers with the "new latest thing" (which really isn't new) and emphasize the hype and trivialize cosmetic procedures and products to a sophomoric level. I read through many magazines and newspapers on a regular basis because I want to see what the public is reading. Almost all articles I've read in the lay media are basically infomercials. I have brochures in my office from companies that are less of a sales job than what I read in magazine articles.

Television is even worse. In a longer show format, they may take more than 40 hours of filming and edit down to a half hour segment which is unrecognizable due to the need to present complex information in short bites. In a short news segment, they will spend at least 10 <u>hours</u> or more filming and edit down to 10 <u>minutes</u> or less of airtime. And most people will only listen to the first couple of minutes.

The media is just as susceptible as patients are to hype and false advertising. The reporter working on a story has no more knowledge than the average patient and has great difficulty judging who or what is credible. Often, the media is unduly influenced by a doctor offering free services or possessing qualities that have nothing to do with credibility or legitimacy. For example, the reporter may be dazzled by the physician's charm, good looks, being a socialite, going to the right events and shindigs to rub elbows with media types and celebrities, etc.

I suspect that many magazine articles are written by reporters and editors who live in New York City because they have high preference for doctors who live in Manhattan who provide them with free services. I'll read many articles that quote a doctor who doesn't have any real expertise in lasers talking about their newest laser procedure and it will be so over hyped with none of the caveats that would be truly vital for readers to know. I'll find out later that the doctor in the article happens to given free treatments to the editor or reporter in order to appear in the magazine. It is quite distressing for me to discover that many physicians have performed quid pro quo deals for exchange of services in order to woo and entice the media for appearances in magazines and TV shows. The reason this is considered unethical is because the media give the false appearance that the article or TV show is done in an unbiased manner. And they do not disclose the secret deal that occurred behind the scenes that was the true motivation for the so-called news piece. So it's not really news and it's certainly not unbiased.

The media should disclose outright if there was any exchange of services for the physician to appear on the show. It seems almost impossible to enforce this, however, because there are so many "winkwink" deals made under the table and all parties involved would deny any culpability.

I know of one example where a certain prominent dermatologist in Manhattan who appears on a national TV news show on a regular basis has a close relationship with the producers and personalities on the show for whom the dermatologist gives regular free services. They have never disclosed this relationship on the show when this dermatologist appears. They say they have this dermatologist appear because of his expertise in the field. However, I have heard this dermatologist speak of many topics that he has no real knowledge of. For example, he spoke about a laser he had just purchased as if he were a laser expert, whereas I knew he had never touched a laser before this recent purchase. He was using his patients as guinea pigs and he was using the media to give him a free promo in order to attract new patients to his practice.

A local news show which features new medical innovations often has the buddies or cronies of the newscaster appear to speak about these topics. This particular show never asks the "true experts" their advice on new innovations, only the same old usual suspects. Once again, a free promo done as a favor.

Many media personalities may brag that they go to the "best" doctor and that's who they ask to be on their shows. I would truly be impressed if the media person actually paid for all their treatments and wasn't getting them free.

Sometimes they quote true experts in the field but the information seems so watered down that I can't believe the physician quoted actually said those things. Low and behold, I will find out from the physician later that he or she was taken out of context and didn't recognize their own statements. I also have had that experience on many occasions.

My local ABC news airs frequent segments hosted by Dr. Dean Edell covering a variety of "breaking" medical stories. Recently he spoke about laser treatments where he labeled two doctors as "laser specialists". What he failed to mention was that one was a family practitioner and the other was a vascular surgeon. The first segment with the family practitioner was about laser hair removal. After interviewing patients, discussing technology, and interviewing the "laser specialist" family practitioner, Dr. Dean Edell and the news announcer warned the public that they should see a dermatologist for laser hair removal because of the complications seen from people who had been treated at salons. They never clarified that the "expert" interviewed was not a dermatologist. Very misleading. Another story that aired a few weeks later featured the Titan device and showed a woman with significant sagging of the neck. She spoke about how she had great results from the Titan. They failed to show any before pictures of her and it was obvious that she still had a lot of sagging. The doctor interviewed could barely put together a coherent statement about what the Titan did. They then showed him standing over an assistant performing the treatment—he didn't even do the treatments himself. Again, he was identified only as a "laser specialist" without any mention of his true specialty -- vascular surgery. A doctor's training and true specialty can easily be ascertained just by looking up their credentials on the AMA or California Medical Board websites. You may ask why the media can't even be bothered to take the extra step of asking what the doctor's specialty is? Well the truth probably is that they either knew he was a vascular surgeon (and the other doctor a family practitioner) and wanted to make him sound more credible to fit the needs of there segment, or they were truly ignorant and did not do any journalistic research. It is possible that they believed him when he sold himself as a "laser specialist". Either way, shame on them. A real "laser expert" has formalized university training – they do not rely on weekend courses, laser company seminars, membership in organizations with misleading names, or convention classes as their sole claim to "expert" status.

An increasing number of media stories won't even bother to find real "experts" in the field. I have heard of many media venues that use doctors because of the publicists that they have hired. These publicists' sole function is to promote these doctors in order to get them on these shows. Some doctors pay publicists $10,000 to $20,000 a month to get their name or spa mentioned in the news and magazines. Most shows I watch on TV seem to be promo pieces and infomercials rather than true news stories. Very few local or national news stories about cosmetic laser surgery highlight doctors who have done anything of real note—they're almost always puff pieces. The fact that a local news show labels anyone as a "laser specialist" who has not proven themselves as such, shows their lack of respect for the field. They're giving the message that basically any doctor qualifies as a "laser specialist" as long as he calls himself one.

I have never hired a publicist or used an agency. I am often asked how I get so many media appearances. Doctors often ask me, "Who's your publicist?" They seem very surprised when I tell them that I don't have one. The next question is always, "Then how did you get in such and such magazine?" I'm always a little shy to say that it's due to my credentials and research and work that got me into those magazines— that I have been called upon because of my true expertise in the field.

I have never appeared in the media because of personal favors. I have never traded services with any individual in order to get in the media. I do not even have a public relations agency or firm working for me. I get quoted in the media purely based upon my knowledge and expertise in the field, and being recognized as a thought leader.

It's also important to be aware of some unethical referral arrangements that exist between some businesses. Some beauticians and aestheticians working in spas and salons refer all their clientele to certain doctors because of "kickbacks" or personal favors (i.e., free services for their staff members, gifts, commissions, etc.). Laser procedures, like other medical treatments, should be referred to practitioners who are the most qualified, not based on commissions.

There are, of course, many ethical beauticians and aestheticians who refer clients to doctors simply because of respect for their skills and expertise. Unfortunately, it's almost impossible to ascertain if there's impropriety occurring in these arrangements. I would be suspicious, however, if a particular salon kept referring to a doctor who is not known for being an expert in that field. For example, there are some beauty salons in my area who refer exclusively to a certain family practitioner who just started performing laser procedures a few years ago and is a true "dabbler". They don't refer clients to the several qualified physicians in the Bay Area. I've heard that this family practitioner constantly invites them to seminars and sends them gift baskets and gift certificates for free services.

I would be equally suspicious of businesses that referred patients with severe heart conditions to a family practitioner instead of a cardiologist.

I rarely give complementary treatments even as a professional courtesy because I don't want to be seen as bribing someone for referrals. I believe that other professionals should refer their patients to me because they respect my skills, not because I offered them free services. I am proud to say that the doctors and their spouses and staff who come to see me pay for their treatments. The people who get free treatments at my office are those who volunteer to be in laser clinical research studies.

Beware of the doctor who tries to sell you on their laser rather than their skill or training. Remember that no one laser can do it all. Also, some lasers may have some side effects which can be easily removed by other lasers. If you're getting laser treatments, wouldn't you want to be in the best hands with access to the widest variety of lasers so that if you did have an adverse effect from one laser, the doctor could adequately treat that side effect with other lasers? If you had a side effect with a doctor who only possesses one laser, then there's no way they can help you with certain side effects that may inevitably result no matter how careful they are.

REFERENCES

1   Lee MWC. "Combination 532-nm and 1064-nm lasers for non-invasive skin rejuvenation and toning." Archives of Dermatology. 2003; 32: 405-412.

2   Lee MWC. "Combination visible and infrared lasers for skin rejuvenation." Seminars in Cutaneous Medicine and Surgery. 2002; 21: 288-300.

3   Zelickson BD, Kilmer SL, Bernstein E, et al. "Pulsed dye laser for sun damaged skin." Lasers Surg Med 1999; 25: 229-36.

CHAPTER 7:

NEW IS NOT
NECESSARILY BETTER

EVERY FEW MONTHS THERE'S the launch of a new laser device from a company that promises to be the new and better kid on the block. Consumers are used to upgrading their lasers and upgrading their cars. They often assume that the "newer" laser must be better.

There are different categories of lasers (i.e., pulsed dye laser, Q-switched Nd:YAG laser, long-pulsed Nd:YAG laser, etc.) (see Chapter 2 for a complete review of lasers) and within each category there are different competing brands. For example, Candela makes several different types of pulsed dye lasers, each with different characteristics or parameters. One Candela pulsed dye laser model may have different spot sizes and different fluences or energy levels than another Candela pulsed dye laser model. Cynosure also makes several different models of pulsed dye lasers. The Cynosure pulsed dye lasers have individual variations from one another, and they in turn have individual variations from the Candela pulsed dye lasers.

Sometimes a "new" laser is simply an upgraded version of the pre-existing older model. There are several different generations of pulsed dye lasers within the Candela family. They are best known for developing and refining the pulsed dye laser and are continually striving to improve and refine this particular technology. This is analogous to upgrading a personal computer on a yearly basis. Every year, there's a newer and faster version of a particular computer model. The newer model usually has different bells and whistles, sometimes better, but not always better than the preexisting one.

Less often, the "new" laser really is actually a brand new technology for which there is no comparison. When the first carbon dioxide (CO2) laser was released on the market, it truly was a technological breakthrough. The first hair removal laser on the market was the ruby laser called the Epilaser released by Palomar in 1998.

The first lasers used for dermatology in the mid to late 1960's emitted a continuous wave, but this was not practical for hair removal, since the beam could not be controlled well enough to avoid collateral skin damage. The development of the Q-switch (similar to a camera shutter) allowed laser energy to be emitted in controlled pulses.

As with electrolysis, the early published clinical data on laser removal involved the successful treatment of ingrown eyelashes.[1] This led to research and even a commercial attempt at a device using an argon (yellow) laser for general market hair removal. This device was rushed to market without adequate testing of effectiveness, and it turned out to be tedious to use and ineffective for permanent hair removal.

Other researchers began using lasers for dermatological procedures and found them useful for removing some kinds of tattoos and for the treatment of some kinds of vascular lesions. In some instances, it was observed that hair loss occurred in treated areas, which led to experiments in epilation in animal models and later human subjects in the early 1990's.

In 1995, one century after the discovery of x-rays, FDA cleared the first laser for hair removal in the U.S., the SoftLight™ Nd:YAG by ThermoLase.[2] This device was rushed to market without adequate testing of effectiveness. It was marketed illegally as painless and permanent until FDA stepped in. It uses a carbon-based lotion as a chromophore (light-absorbing molecule). This lotion was rubbed into the skin following waxing, with the hope it would penetrate into the hair follicle. The laser would then rapidly heat the carbon, causing a shock wave of energy that had the potential to damage nearby cells. This process was found to be more complicated and less effective than targeting chromophores that occur naturally in the skin (i.e., melanin which is the pigment in the skin).

The device was sold to physicians and treatments were offered in a chain of proprietary clinics called Spa Thira, primarily in affluent communities. Consumers basically paid to be guinea pigs. By the time a medical paper appeared in 1997 which observed full regrowth of all hair[3], consumers had already spent hundreds of thousands of dollars on treatments. They quickly shifted their marketing strategy away from permanent hair removal to a "hair-management strategy," but word was beginning to get out.

In 1998, a class action lawsuit was brought against the company by a consumer alleging ThermoLase "advertised SoftLight laser hair removal as long lasting with the knowledge that such treatments did not achieve that result."[4] ThermoLase quietly settled out of court later that year. In 1999, following other lawsuits and an annual loss of over $41 million, they began closing or selling their spas.[5] In 2000, with the stock down 92% from its high, ThermoLase was folded back into its parent company, which no longer manufactures or markets SoftLight in the U.S.

In 1997, the FDA cleared several types of devices that claimed to remove hair by targeting melanin in the hair. As with the earlier devices, these devices were rushed to market without adequate testing of effectiveness.

Incremental improvement in equipment since 1997, such as more ergonomically-designed handpieces and methods of skin cooling, have made treatment generally more tolerable and reduce the likelihood of some side effects. The publication of clinical observations have also led to more optimized treatment parameters, but understanding of lasers and their long-term effects on hair and other skin structures is still in the early stages.

For effective hair removal to occur, the follicle (the bulb, to be specific) which is located deep within the skin has to be reached and destroyed by the laser beam. Destruction occurs when a certain threshold of thermal energy (or heat) is delivered to the target. The goal is to destroy the target (hair follicle or blood vessel) without damaging the surrounding skin. In order to accomplish this, several criteria need to be met. First, a wavelength of light specific for the target's chromophore must be selected. That wavelength of light must emit a fluence (heat energy) level that is high is enough and the pulse duration (laser exposure time) must be long enough to destroy the target. The target must be destroyed before causing damage to the surrounding skin. Adequate cooling of the skin is essential to avoid complications such as blistering and burns. Many newer lasers incorporate sophisticated cooling devices. A "new" laser may be a preexisting older technology such as the pulsed dye laser with the addition of a new cooling device. Candela's Vbeam was such an improvement. Older technology with a new spin.

It may be surprising for the consumer to discover that despite all the popularity of laser treatments, there is relatively little good quality scientific research on lasers in medicine. Prescription drugs that are tested and approved for marketing undergo rigorous multicenter testing with thousands of patients followed for several years to monitor the long-term effects of the drugs and associated side effects. Drug companies invest millions of dollars to perform these clinical studies. Compare this to the majority of laser companies who may sponsor one or a few studies consisting of only a few dozen patients who are followed for only 3 to 6 months. Many laser companies sell and promote lasers before they have any studies published at all. It's common to perform a literature search on laser studies and find that most of the studies consist of 5 to 10 patients who received one treatment and were followed for 3 months. This sampling is so insignificant that it seems preposterous to be able to make any definitive conclusions on the safety or efficacy of that treatment. But many laser companies will use a study with 10 or less patients that reports positive results and go running with that study and promote it as if the results from this small sampling could be extrapolated to the whole population.

Laser studies are expensive and slow to perform, analyze, present, and publish. The laser companies are quick to promote their new devices and procedures, even before efficacy and safety are well established, and even before the FDA has given approval. And another important thing to keep in mind is that the FDA is far more concerned with safety than efficacy when it comes to laser devices. Clinical data may show that a laser provides "significant improvement" in cellulite. What qualifies as "significant improvement"? That may be demonstrated through as little as 10 to 20% improvement, sometimes even less.

A blue light used for acne treatment was shown through one study to cause half the patients in the study to have some improvement (anything more than 0%). This means that half the patients had absolutely no improvement at all. Half of the patients that showed improvement had at least 30% improvement. This means that the other half had less than 30% improvement. This study was available for all to read but unfortunately most physicians who bought the device never bothered to read the study. Instead, they chose to the listen to the laser sales rep who would claim the blue light "cleared" acne. The physicians would turn around and run advertisements that claimed they had a revolutionary new device that "cleared" acne. One of the physicians who purchased this new blue light was seen on a local TV news station claiming that he had a brand new laser that would "cure" acne after only one treatment. Of course, this was never proven by any scientific study. And the blue light could never perform to this unrealistic level.

The laser company that produced the blue light used in the acne study ran an advertisement in medical specialty journals and publications that contained the photograph of a model with half of her face with severe acne and the other half of her face was completely clear. Even the casual observer would note that there was something peculiar or artificial about the photo. I knew the make-up artist who told me she was hired by the company for a photo shoot for this particular model in which she was told to apply make-up to make the model appear as if she had severe acne. She was also hired for another photo shoot where she was instructed to paint large veins on a model's leg so that the "before" picture showed the fake veins and the "after" photo was of the model's real leg without any veins. Incidentally, this make-up artist also did a lot of work for films requiring special effects.

The largest body of work exists in the area of laser hair removal. Even so, well-controlled prospective studies are lacking. Although the amount of unwanted hair in a treated area can be effectively diminished, it is unclear if complete elimination of unwanted hair from any anatomic area can be achieved with any of the existing laser systems. Given the current available information, it seems unlikely that 100% permanent hair reduction can ever be achieved no matter what laser system is used.

Because lasers are usually rushed to market without a full understanding of their capabilities and limitations, it's vital that researchers, practitioners, and consumers continue to make their experiences known to the public.

In my practice, I have more than 25 lasers and have worked with many more lasers than that. Through the course of my residency and fellowship training and practice, I have worked with almost every laser there is on the market and am familiar with most of the existent lasers. I am constantly researching new lasers and working with laser companies to help develop and refine existent and new emerging technology and procedures. I am probably 2 to 3 years ahead of the learning curve, meaning that I know about most lasers 2 to 3 years before other doctors or consumers ever hear of them. Being literally at the cutting edge and forefront of my field, I have the advantage of testing out lasers well ahead of the curve, and am able to decide early on if that laser is going to be advantageous to my patients. I test many lasers for different companies and help them with clinical studies. I know from direct experience whether the laser is really effective and safe. After the study is finished, I only keep the lasers that I feel are advantageous for my patients. My patients benefit by having a physician who is very knowledgeable about any given laser and they have the benefit of always having access to the latest and best technology. If there's a newer better laser, I'll be the first one to get it. If after testing a new laser, I determine that it's not what it's cracked up to be, I decide not to offer it to my patients. Many times my patients will ask if I heard of a new laser they read about in a magazine. The answer always is yes, but then I often have to explain to them why I decided not to get that laser for my practice. It's usually because it didn't perform better than a preexisting laser and it didn't offer any advantage over another laser that I already have. The bottom line in my practice is that I want to offer the patient the best treatment available. Patients may request a certain device that I do possess but it may not be the best treatment for the condition they want to treat, so I direct them towards another device that will provide better results.

I probably have more than 50 studies that I have finished or am in the process of finishing that I haven't had time to publish. Many physicians have performed studies of high quality that they haven't gotten around to publish yet. This is unfortunate for the public and the medical community because they would really benefit from these studies. The fact is that laser technology is a rapidly evolving new field with a constant onslaught of new devices and procedures that take time to study and examine thoroughly, and even more time to construct and publish a meaningful scientific paper. Physicians who want to conduct thorough research, such as myself, find it difficult if not reprehensible to rush out studies just to be published without having done due diligence. I believe there are a large number of publications that were rushed to press simply for the sake of being published first without regard to the quality of the scientific work that was performed. And many of these rushed publications make hasty conclusions that have not held out with the test of time. If they had been thoroughly conducted with a large sample size (several hundred subjects) and proper controls and proper long-term follow-up (over 1 to 2 years), many of the conclusions would be far different.

Patient participation in clinical studies is vital for the advancement of science and medicine. However, patient safety is paramount in conducting studies. I only participate in studies using devices that have been tested on animal models and found to be safe in humans during preliminary testing. By the time the laser is brought to my practice for clinical trials, I already have considerable knowledge and confidence in the laser's safety and performance before establishing parameters for a prospectively controlled study for which we enroll human volunteers. I'm very careful about not doing anything which could cause harm to a patient during any clinical study. I would rather sacrifice some efficacy over any compromises in safety. In other words, I wouldn't push the treatment settings to get better results if I thought there would be any chance of causing complications. But some researchers have a rather blasé attitude towards their research subjects and really see them as guinea pigs. I hear some researchers actually brag about how many human subjects that they've burned or scarred during studies.

Research aside, it's more important what I recommend to my paying customers. Fraxel™ is the best example of how a new laser is not necessarily better—it's just different. I tested the Fraxel two years ago and was not impressed. It had been hyped up to be "better than the CO2 laser with no downtime". In actuality, it produced results inferior to the CO2 and Erbium lasers, had comparable downtime to the Erbium, and was a lot more expensive than the CO2 or Erbium lasers. So in the end, I could not justify adding this laser to my practice.

In response to criticisms about the unimpressive results, it has been proposed to turn up the settings with the Fraxel so that it actually causes a wound more similar to the CO2 laser in order to get better wrinkle reduction, but then the downtime is comparable to the CO2. By turning up the settings of the Fraxel™, it becomes a truly invasive procedure (like the CO2) instead of a semi-invasive procedure. If that's the case, why not go ahead and just do CO2 resurfacing? Conversely, I have the same capabilities to turn down the settings with the CO2 laser or Erbium laser in order to mimic the Fraxel laser to perform a semi-invasive procedure—why would a physician buy another expensive device just to do what they can already do better with one of their existing lasers? The Fraxel™ truly is a laser in search of an indication.

Another void in the laser scientific literature is the absence of negative studies that are often withheld from publication. Often, the negative studies would be far more meaningful for physicians and patients to discern if a particular laser treatment is effective or worth investing money in, but there are many disincentives to publishing negative data. Many physicians and researchers have working relationships with various laser companies and don't want to endanger these relationships with negative studies that could potentially harm a company's reputation or stock value. Some physicians only conduct studies that are being funded by laser companies, and companies won't pay to have negative studies published.

The term "permanent hair removal" is itself a misnomer. One would think that permanent hair removal constitutes complete 100% removal of all hairs without ever having regrowth. If using this definition, no such thing exists. It's all a fairytale—give it up and go home. In general, when the FDA gives clearance for a laser to deliver "permanent hair removal", they're referring to a laser's ability to eliminate hair growth for a given period of time, usually about 6 months. There are no standardized terminology or performance standards for hair removal.

The lack of an industry consensus on what constitutes permanent hair removal has caused great confusion for consumers.

Most effective hair removal devices are capable of reducing unwanted pigmented hairs and slowing down hair growth to the point that there may be a relatively "hair-free period" that lasts from 4 to 6 months. The hairs that grow back tend to be lighter and finer and grow slower. This is called the "miniaturization" of hairs.

There have been several generations of hair removal devices. The first generation consisted of the ruby laser (Epilaser, Palomar) which is well-absorbed by melanin (chromophore containing pigment). The problem with this laser was that it would be so well-absorbed by melanin that it would be absorbed by the melanin in the skin and not just the melanin contained in the hair follicle. The incidence of burns with this particular laser was much higher, even in the whitest skin. It was contraindicated for use in tan and darker skin.

The second generation of hair removal lasers consisted of the 810 nm diode laser (LightSheer, Coherent now Lumenis) which received FDA clearance in 1999 and the 755 nm alexandrite laser (GentleLase, Candela) which are extremely effectively and safe at targeting darker hairs in white skin patients. The margin of safety was much narrower for tan and darker skin. Even though the companies attempted to market these lasers for all skin types, it turned out that there were greater complications in tan and darker skin patients.

In 2000, an intense pulsed light device received FDA clearance for hair removal (Epilight, ESC). Unlike a laser which is a single wavelength of high intensity light, an intense pulsed light device is a broad band of light containing multiple wavelengths which are nonspecific, scattered and much more diffuse.

The third generation of hair removal devices helped to address tan and darker skin patients with the advent of the long-pulsed Nd:YAG 1064 nm lasers. There were several companies who came out with similar devices around the same time but Altus (now Cutera) was the first to get FDA clearance in 2001. Laserscope got FDA clearance for the Lyra a month later. The earlier long-pulsed Nd:YAG lasers include the CoolGlide (Altus now Cutera), Lyra (Laserscope)(current version is the Gemini), and Profile (Sciton).

More recently Candela developed an Nd:YAG laser safe for darker skin called the GentleYAG since their primary hair removal laser, the GentleLase (alexandrite laser) is less desirable for use on darker skin. This was largely in response to the need to have a laser safe for dark skin since the long-pulsed Nd:YAG became the gold standard for performing hair removal in tan and darker skin. The GentleLase has the additional problem of actually causing increased hair growth when used on darker skin patients. That's because the user would turn down the fluence (energy) level in order to decrease the chance of causing burns in the darker skin patient. Delivering lower energy levels would actually stimulate hair growth instead of destroying the hair follicles.

New technology may be better…or not. Is "new improved" Tide™ really new and improved? Some older lasers that did not do well when they first came out on the market get repackaged and marketed as a "new laser". The company is counting on physicians and the public having a short memory so that they don't remember that the "new" Epilight is an intense pulsed light device similar to the "old" Photoderm which got nicknamed the "Photoburn" because there were so many complications.

Chemical peels are notorious for being reinvented every few years as the "latest and greatest innovation". Chemical peels have been around since the time of the early Egyptians who were using it to lighten their skin centuries ago. Every few years I'll see a "groundbreaking" report on the local news station with local physician promoting the "newest breakthrough" in cosmetic surgery and it turns out to be a chemical peel named something else to make it sound new. A few years ago there was a craze about the "blue peel" by Obagi which is actually a chemical peel. It contains the same acid that's been used for years in traditional chemical peels. The only difference was Obagi added a blue color indicator that would alert the practitioner that the peel was done whereas the traditional chemical peel turns a frosted white color to indicate that it's done. There was a great deal of marketing and promotion to make this peel sound extraordinary and revolutionary. Not to say that the peel wasn't effective, it just wasn't unique.

Another procedure called the Exoderm™ was developed in Israel and adopted by American physicians. It's a chemical peel and produces similar results as other chemical peels. But it's constantly being promoted as being "like a facelift" and a "groundbreaking new procedure" to make the consumer think it's something new and different. Not that there's anything wrong with chemical peels—they do work. But just don't be fooled by the "new and improved" because it's really the same as it ever was.

Mesotherapy is another example of a procedure that gets revamped every few years as the "new hot thing" but it's been around for over 50 years. The problem with mesotherapy is that there haven't been any well-controlled studies performed and most of the claims have not been substantiated by scientific evidence. Mesotherapy involves the injections of multiple cocktails containing various ingredients ranging from phosphatidylcholine (a preservative purported to dissolve fat), antioxidants, vitamins, and other purported anti-aging ingredients. Mesotherapy is the best example of human experimentation because it's being done without any data on its safety and efficacy to support its use. Most physicians would admit freely that they don't know what mesotherapy does. It's an alchemist's cave. Those who perform mesotherapy make wild claims about melting away fat and cellulite but when asked to present evidence or studies to support their claims, they are not able to produce it. In 2003, the Brazilian National Agency of Health banned the use of phosphatidylcholine, which is the main ingredient used in most mesotherapy procedures, due to lack of scientific data. Meanwhile, medical societies and organizations in the U.S. caution doctors that further studies to determine efficacy, safety, and mechanism of action need to be performed before this technique can be endorsed.

Until the science catches up with the technology and there is more availability of well-controlled studies in peer-reviewed journals, the consumer has to be aware of the rampant hype that exists in the mainstream press, promotional materials produced by manufacturers and practitioners, and unreliable anecdotal reports from consumers. Many consumer websites are just knowledgeable enough to be dangerous. I hope the information in this book will help the consumer maneuver through the hype.

References

1. Berry J. Recurrent trichiasis: treatment with laser photocoagulation. Ophthalmic Surgery. 1979 Jul; 10(7):36-8.

2. FDA Docket K950019. 5 April 1995.

3. Nanni CA, Alster TS. Optimizing treatment parameters for hair removal using a topical carbon-based solution and 1064-nm Q-switched neodymium:YAG laser energy. Archives of Dermatology. 1997 Dec;133(12):1546-9.

4. Tester v. ThermoLase, Calif. Superior Court (S.F. County, case #995285).

5. TLZ 1998 Annual Report and SEC 10K, 18 December 1998.

CHAPTER 8:

BEST RESULTS ARE ACHIEVED BY COMBINING MULTIPLE MODALITIES

PATIENTS OFTEN COME TO my office seeking the fountain of youth and more beautiful skin. They ask me what they can do to have better skin. Often the answer is to combine multiple procedures to achieve the best results. Patients who follow my recommendations get the best results. Some patients don't like what they hear and will shop around until they find someone who will tell them what they want to hear even if it's not true.

My front office staff keeps me apprised of the types of questions that are asked on phone call inquiries. It's amazing to me how many people call the office asking about prices only and nothing else. They don't care about the doctor's training or qualifications. In fact, they don't even bother to ask if the doctor does the treatments. The most frequently asked question is, "How much do you charge for Botox™?" Sometimes their response to the answer is, "Did you know I can get that for half the price?" And when the staff member asks them where, they'll inevitably say it's a salon or beauty parlor where the injection isn't administered by a doctor (and probably grossly diluted or possibly even "fake" Botox™). They don't seem to care that they're comparing apples and oranges. You can't compare a board-certified dermatologist with advanced fellowship training in performing Botox™ with a nurse or aesthetician working at a salon unsupervised who has questionable training if any. Same with lasers and any other cosmetic procedure.

Purchasing a cosmetic service performed by an expert physician is not like purchasing a refrigerator or car. You can shop around for a Whirlpool refrigerator by calling different stores for the lowest price and you'll get the same refrigerator no matter what you pay. The same does not hold for cosmetic procedures. These are services, not commodities. The service is only as good as the person performing it. Could you expect a layperson to paint the Sistine Chapel as well as Michelangelo?

If you called 10 different offices and got similar prices ranging from $450 to $550 for a procedure from 9 of the offices and then the 10th office gave you a price of $250 for the same procedure, wouldn't you logically conclude that there must be something wrong? Or would you think that you had found the bargain of the century? Even if it were a refrigerator, I would still be suspicious that there was some hidden risk that you're not being made aware of. For cosmetic procedures, the lowest price that is so far off from everyone else would truly, without a doubt, indicate that something is amiss. You probably get what you pay for. And if something sounds too good to be true, it is.

Some doctors and salons outright lie. Some just don't know what they're talking about. They're not intentionally lying but just ignorant. Laser companies oftentimes over hype their lasers and doctors just repeat the company line, not realizing it's not true. They learn the hard way after many patients come back complaining that the treatment didn't work the way it was promised. Sometimes the laser is not at fault, only the practitioner who's overselling it is.

It's common to see ads in the newspaper for laser hair removal at salons for $99 or less. There are even some places (usually illegal) that will advertise free laser treatments just to get people to go in. A tattoo parlor in my local area runs ads in the "Pennysaver," which is a classified rag that runs free ads ranging from garage sales to cries from the lovelorn, advertising free laser treatments without any mention of who is doing the treatment or what is the name of the business, and there's only the address and phone number. It's an obvious ploy to get people to come in so that the customer will sign up for other paid procedures. Also, there's no disclosure that hair removal requires multiple treatments so only the first treatment is free. Same with the laser hair removal salons that run ads for $99 or less. They don't mention that you'll have to do a lot of treatments and that for each subsequent treatment you'll have to purchase a package of 6 or more treatments for $2,000 to $3,000. And that's just the beginning. Then you soon find out that since this salon doesn't know what they're doing, the laser treatments aren't working at all so you basically threw away $3,000. And since many of these places are operating shoddy businesses, they'll often close down and run away with all the money from prepaid packages before they even had to deliver on the services agreed upon.

I often hear people complain about how their laser treatments didn't work and they blame it on the laser. They should blame it on the operator of the laser instead. Most likely the wrong laser was used or the operator wasn't properly trained so they couldn't optimize the treatment or they weren't properly educating the patient on what to expect.

The most common complaints I hear regarding laser treatments are as follows:

1. *The blood vessel on my nose didn't go away after one treatment:*

    Possible reasons:
    1a. The wrong device was used. If an intense pulsed light (IPL) (also known as the "FotoFacial" was used, it's possible that the vessel wouldn't even clear after 20 treatments. (See Chapter 2 for further elaboration on why).

    1b. Even if the correct laser was used, not enough treatments were performed. If the doctor told you that the vessel would be guaranteed to be completely gone after only one treatment, then the doctor (or nurse) was either intentionally lying or just plain ignorant.

1c. Even if the proper treatment was performed the proper number of times, the blood vessel could recur. No one should ever promise you that a particular blood vessel can never recur. Sometimes it's not a true recurrence, it's actually a new blood vessel. The important point to make is that there will be future blood vessels that will need to be treated and that does not indicate a failure of the first series of treatments. Most lesions require a series of treatments followed by periodic maintenance treatments to keep under control. The same applies for pigmented lesions such as freckles and age spots.

2. *This freckle (or blood vessel) I had treated came back:*

Possible reasons:

2a. You should have been informed that any lesion can recur or you could develop new lesions. Freckles and broken capillaries on the face are often caused by sun damage. Most people get a lot of sun damage just with daily living and driving the car. Even wearing sunscreen doesn't prevent recurrence of these lesions (it does slow them down though, so keep wearing sunscreen!).

2b. Blood vessels around the sides of the nose can occur from frequent blowing of the nose and rubbing. They are the most resistant to treatment and recur the fastest.

2c. Being on hormones or pregnancy can cause increased darkening of pigmented lesions. Due to hormonal stimulation, freckles or other pigmented lesions may be resistant to treatment or they may recur very quickly or even get worse after treatment. I recommend that the patient try to get off hormones before undergoing certain laser treatments. Also, it may be a waste of money to undergo a series of expensive laser treatments to remove pigmentation if you're planning to get pregnant soon. The brown spots will likely get worse while pregnant so you should wait until after pregnancy to get them removed.

3. How come my best friend Mary Lou's blood vessel went away after one treatment and mine didn't?

Possible reasons:

3a. No, this doesn't mean that Mary Lou had a more brilliant doctor and you had a moron treat you. It's amazing how many people have friends with mythical results (kind of like the big fish that everyone seems to be able to catch except you)—total clearance of hair after one treatment, total removal of every blemish after one treatment, total clearance of leg veins after one treatment, etc. There are some <u>rare</u> circumstances that a blood vessel may clear after one treatment but it's usually a smaller one and it also depends on the location. I have had some patients with blood vessels clear after one treatment but they're the rare exception, not the norm. I would never suggest that this would be an expected occurrence. Like the rest of life, there is a great bell-shaped curve when it comes to results from cosmetic procedures. It is the job of the responsible physician to properly educate the patient to establish realistic expectations, and that means also giving the worst case scenario. I could sign up 100% of patients who come in for consults for procedures if I promised them the moon. In the end, 1 out of 10 patients would be thrilled and the other 9 would be very disappointed.

3b. I would question whether the friend even had the same condition as you. After further questioning, I may discover that the patient's friend had a light small freckle which cleared after one treatment whereas the patient has a multitude of much thicker and larger liver spots. Or that the friend had a small tiny capillary and the patient has very large veins. But in the conversation they equate them to be the same. Friends usually don't examine each other's before and after photos for clinical accuracy and diagnosis during their discussions.

An analogous situation occurs with acne. Many teenagers tell me their best friend cleared up with Retin-A so how come they have to go on Accutane? The answer usually is that their friend had very mild acne whereas the patient has severe nodulocystic acne which is leaving a lot of scars behind and responds usually only to Accutane.

4. *My friend had much better results than I did:*

Possible reasons:

4a. I've often had patients who know each other compare results. A common scenario is Patient A says that Patient B's skin looks much better. In this case, Patient B did CO2 laser resurfacing and Patient A did microdermabrasion. Not even comparing the same procedures!

4b. Patient A may have combined multiple procedures and Patient A only did one procedure.

4c. There's a big difference in the skin quality prior to treatment. Patient B may have less sun damage than Patient A so that the final result also looks much better.

4d. There's an age disparity. A difference of 10 years can also be reflected in the final results. Someone with deep wrinkles may not get as dramatic an effect as someone with moderate wrinkles, depending on the procedure.

5. *I went to a doctor with a great reputation but the laser treatment didn't turn out well:*

Possible reasons:

5a. The doctor you went to may be famous for breast implants or face-lifts but perhaps just learned how to use lasers last week and just bought a new laser and this is a new toy for him. An A+ doctor in plastic surgery may not be an A+ doctor for lasers.

5b. The doctor may be a famous dermatologist but has limited knowledge about lasers. He may have theoretical knowledge about lasers and sound like he knows what he's talking about but doesn't have practical experience with lasers and only owns a few lasers or rents them. He's an A+ dermatologist but <u>not</u> an A+ laser surgeon.

5c. The doctor is an A+ laser surgeon but for whatever reason doesn't own the A+ lasers. Perhaps he purchased certain lasers because of cost and timing and hasn't been able to update them, so meanwhile he's forced to use substandard lasers.

5d. Maybe the laser treatment turned out as best as it could but either the doctor didn't take the time to educate you properly about what to expect, or you didn't listen.

This last point highlights the necessity of not only finding a qualified physician but also finding one with whom you can establish rapport and trust. The best laser surgeon in the world cannot help you if they are not willing to take the time to listen or properly communicate with you or vice versa. I have had patients come in for consultation who were so rushed that they shortchanged themselves from getting proper advice. I am constantly astonished at patients who sabotage themselves. I was willing to give the patient as much time as they needed, but they couldn't sit still long enough to listen to the answers. So, if you are fortunate enough to find a doctor who is willing to take time to talk to you, you had best give them your undivided attention!

6. *I had several FotoFacial (intense pulsed light) treatments and it didn't help my wrinkles or scars:*

Possible reasons:

6a. The wrong device was used if that was the problem you were trying to treat. The IPL device does not help with wrinkles or scars (see Chapter 2 for review of lasers).

6b. Even with CO_2 laser resurfacing which would be the most effective treatment for wrinkles and for some types of scarring, there will never be complete resolution of the problem. Even the best laser in the best practitioner's hands would not produce 100% removal of wrinkles or scars. It's not physiologically possible. It's realistic to expect great improvement (60 to 70% improvement is common for wrinkle reduction with CO_2 laser) but don't expect to look 20 if you're 65 years old. Most people think they look at least 10 to 15 years younger after CO_2 laser resurfacing.

6c. You can get some reduction of wrinkles and scars with noninvasive lasers but the best results can be achieved by combining multiple modalities. For example, combining a laser that stimulates collagen such as the Nd:YAG (Lyra, Gemini, CoolGlide, Varia, Profile) or diode (SmoothBeam, Polaris) laser combined with a device capable of deep thermal heating such as the ThermaCool (Thermage) can provide excellent results with no downtime. Adding an additional laser such as the Erbium:YAG (used at a low fluence level) which can do less invasive resurfacing than the CO2 laser with much less downtime can further optimize the results.

For treatment of difficult problems such as striae (stretchmarks) and scars, I combine multiple devices to achieve the best results. For example, for acne scarring, I will often combine several different non-invasive lasers to maximize collagen remodeling which would help "plump" up the skin below depressed scars. Adding the KTP laser would help reduce brown and red discolorations often associated with scarring. Adding the ThermaCool would help tighten the skin which would make scars look better. Adding the Erbium:YAG laser would help smooth out the irregularities on the surface of the skin. This is called the "3-D Approach" which addresses each layer of skin from superficial to deep. In the end, I will have used at least 7 to 8 different devices to optimize the results. In addition, fillers (such as Restylane®, Collagen®, Cosmoderm®, Hylaform®, Captique®, Sculptra®, etc.) may be used for deep scars and craters.

For stretch marks, I also combine multiple devices to achieve the best results. Since stretch marks are defects of the collagen similar to scars, they respond to many of the same treatments that scars do. I combine several different noninvasive lasers to maximize collagen remodeling to help "plump" up the atrophic (depressed and thinned out) skin. Adding the KTP or pulsed dye lasers help reduce red or purple discolorations. Adding the UVB laser (ReLume or Excimer) helps with hypopigmented (white) stretchmarks. Adding the ThermaCool helps to tighten the skin which makes stretchmarks look better. Adding a device such as the VelaSmooth (Syneron) uses three forms of energy (optical light, bipolar radiofrequency, mechanical manipulation) which can also help with some skin contouring. In the end, I may have used at least 8 to 9 different devices to optimize the results.

Rosacea is best treated with multiple modalities such as combining intense pulsed light with KTP or pulsed dye laser and long-pulsed Nd: YAG laser (see Chapter 2 for review of lasers). But unless somebody owned all of these lasers, they could not offer the best combination of treatments, and also would not be able to afford to rent several different lasers and offer the combination treatments to you at a reasonable price.

The reason that I can afford to offer multiple lasers to treat a particular condition is that I have all the lasers in my possession and I basically do volume discounts. I can decide to add on a 2nd, 3rd, or 4th laser in order to optimize treatments results and thereby give the patient "more bang for the buck" and not have the price reflect exactly how much value they're getting. For example, I may treat a patient with rosacea with 3 different devices: IPL and KTP and long-pulsed Nd: YAG lasers. I will charge $750 for one treatment utilizing all 3 devices which also would require 3 times the amount of time required for using 1 device. Another physician may charge $750 for using only one device, the KTP laser. If the patient went to that physician and asked what it would cost for getting all 3 devices, that physician may have to charge $750 x 3 = $2,250 in order to perform a treatment using all 3 devices. Even if that physician were charging less for the one laser, let's say the charge is $500 for the KTP laser, the patient is still getting far less in the end for their money.

Using the large handpiece of an IPL device serves some purposes—it is able to treat large areas at a time and does help treat the "background blush" although it's incapable of treating discrete lesions. Combining the IPL with lasers allows the practitioner to perform the treatment in a more expeditious manner therefore keeping the price reasonable. For example, doing 3 to 4 passes with the IPL will help to decrease the number of passes that need to be performed with the KTP laser. The practitioner needs to "paint" over the entire face (as if painting over an empty canvas and filling all the blank spaces). Painting over the entire face with a small 5 mm round spot takes a lot longer than painting over the face with a 10 to 20 mm rectangular handpiece (however, it does look a little more like "stapling" with a brick—that's where the analogy of a chisel vs. a sledgehammer is quite fitting). The IPL handpiece allows one to cover large areas although it's quite clumsy and lacks finesse. The IPL requires flat surfaces—its large flat surface makes it difficult to treat curved and narrow areas (i.e., nose, around eyes, lips, hands, etc.) The laser handpiece allows one to be precise and controlled and treats lesions of any size and can treat any surface area easily. The laser is the nimble ballerina while the IPL is the heavy sumo wrestler.

The best treatment both in terms of efficacy and expediency involve combining the IPL device with different lasers. I use the IPL device to cover large surface areas and to decrease the total number of passes that will be needed with the KTP laser. I then hone in on individual lesions with the KTP laser, utilizing its power and precision for better results and deeper penetration. The KTP laser is able to treat lesions of any size and depth, on any surface of the body.

If my office burned down and I had to start all over again, the first laser I would acquire would be the KTP laser, the Gemini laser by Laserscope to be specific. It is the dermatologist's best friend. It is the gold standard for treating vascular and pigmented lesions, which is the primary complaint that most patients have.

An artist may prefer one tool above all others—but to create a true masterpiece, the artist will require many tools. This is the same for the experienced laser surgeon.

As a sculptor or builder, I would argue that both a chisel and a sledgehammer are necessary tools to create a masterpiece. It's the way the craftsman uses the tools that ultimately make the difference.

Besides possessing necessary tools of the trade, skill and experience are requisites for good laser treatments because there is no "cook-book" that describes the ideal approach. The "McLaser" model will always fail because it's impossible to take a "boilerplate" approach to mass marketing laser procedures. The rate limiting factor will always be the skill and experience and artistry of the practitioner.

In addition to finding a master laser surgeon who possesses all the necessary criteria to be an A+ doctor and owns all the A+ lasers, you also need to find someone who's willing to take the time to listen to you and find out what you want. Some of the best doctors in the world ultimately don't make their patients happy because they don't take time to listen and to communicate. But keep in mind that this is a two-way street. The best doctor in the world can't help a patient who doesn't communicate with the doctor and is unwilling to take responsibility for their own decisions and actions.

Many a treatment has been sabotaged by the noncompliant patient. This is the kind of patient that all doctors dread. Despite the doctor's best efforts, the noncompliant patient seems intent on being their own worst enemy. This is the patient that never follows the instructions (usually resulting from neglect or carelessness, not from sheer intent) and then blames the doctor when things inevitably don't turn out as planned. I, along with all doctors, have had patients to whom I and my staff provide verbal instructions many times, provide detailed written instructions for them to read and copies to take home, even have them initial the instructions signifying that they have read and understood all the points, and still the patient comes back and has not followed the instructions and claims that "nobody told them". They blame everyone else but themselves. Even when confronted with the written instructions that they initialed, they say, "I didn't read that." When asked if they remembered the verbal instructions, they say, "I didn't hear that."

The worst kind of patient is the one who goes into the doctor saying, "Do whatever you want—I trust you." The doctor may be a genius but is not a mindreader! No two people have the same concept of external beauty. Beauty is truly in the eyes of the beholder. And it is much more important that you look beautiful when you look at yourself in the mirror rather than what the doctor sees. Some of the best results are not perceived as such by the patient. This is very difficult and challenging for both the doctor and the patient. Some people will never be happy, no matter what is done for them. It is important for a doctor to recognize patients who may not psychologically be capable of having realistic expectations and persuade them not to have cosmetic treatments and instead seek psychological counseling.

The doctor can only inform the patient of what the options are and what to realistically expect. There are no guarantees with cosmetic surgery. Lasers can produce wonderful results but it's important to be made aware of the limitations and the possible risks of undergoing laser procedures. A doctor who is willing to take the time to explain things to you and wants to help you make your own decisions is worth their weight in gold.

Once you meet an A+ laser surgeon who owns the A+ lasers, listen to their recommendations carefully. There are all sorts of reasons why one consultation may not provide all the answers. Perhaps you haven't even formulated the questions in your mind. The doctor can only help you if you are able to clearly articulate your needs and priorities. Having done that, the doctor can then recommend a comprehensive treatment plan that will address all of your needs.

It's important to prioritize your needs in order to help you figure out how you're going to finance your procedures. Cosmetic surgical makeovers are very much like home makeovers. Most people don't tackle remodeling the entire house in one fell swoop. They will usually work on one section of the house at a time. Same with cosmetic procedures. You can work with the doctor to help map out a game plan that fits into your budget. But you can only do this effectively if you have the entire map laid out in front of you.

Don't get caught up in the trap of doing a little here and little there. You'll be shocked and dismayed when you discover how much money you end up wasting on a bunch of little things that don't really accomplish anything. I meet so many people who feel like they wasted thousands of dollars on FotoFacials that didn't address any of their problems. They always say to me that they only wish they knew from the beginning that the FotoFacial wasn't the right procedure for them—that they'd rather save up their money for the more expensive laser procedures because that's what they ended up finding out that they needed anyway. If they had only gone to a true laser expert who would take the time to help educate them on all the available options so that they could have the big picture instead of working piecemeal.

Most people instantly realize (on hindsight) that it doesn't make sense to spend thousands of dollars on microdermabrasions and FotoFacials if in the end, you're still going to need the more expensive laser procedures. They would rather have been told that from the beginning so they could allocate their funds towards the more effective treatments. But hindsight is 20-20.

Some people may assume that I would be outrageously priced. I am actually underpriced for what I do. The initial price may sound more expensive, especially if you're comparing it to a treatment being performed by a nurse or aesthetician at a laser chain where there is no proper supervision by a physician or proper training of the staff. But if you break the price down into its proper components, then you realize that I'm actually undercharging for the services.

Another example of how a patient may not be getting the most for their money is the following scenario: the patient goes to a clinic where the IPL treatment (nicknamed "FotoFacial") is being offered for $350. However, the procedure is performed by a nurse who learned to do the procedure the week before by going to a weekend seminar. The nurse goes over the entire face only once and doesn't know how to "spot treat" (this involves going over specific lesions several times with different devices which the IPL cannot reach)(see Chapter 2). The same procedure may cost slightly more at my office but I go over the entire face several times with the IPL device using proper settings (which I would know how to optimize because of my training, experience, and expertise), and would also have the proper devices and know-how to "spot treat" individual lesions which normally would not respond to the IPL device. So in the end, it doesn't matter how much money the patient "saved" by going to the cheaper place, they end up having suboptimal results. In fact, that's why the majority of patients going to places such as I have described end up complaining that these treatments don't work. They have thrown their money away by spending their money on charlatans who have conned them out of their money and they mistakenly blame it on the technology being faulty.

This happens all the time with the Thermage treatment. Nicknamed the "nonsurgical lift", the ThermaCool (Thermage) treatment is very technique dependent. There are some physicians or nurses who perform the treatment in 15 to 30 minutes and only use 100 to 300 pulses on the entire face. In my practice, it takes 2 to 2-1/2 hours to perform a full-face treatment properly using 900 or more pulses. Many patients call around asking for prices not realizing there is such huge variation in the way the procedure is being performed. The lack of uniformity with which this procedure is being performed is why there is great discrepancy in the results patients are reporting. Some patients are getting no results at all, but that is most likely due to the way the procedure was performed.

With regards to Thermage treatments, patients who receive multiple passes done at lower settings get better results with less complications than patients who receive fewer passes done at higher settings. Some warning signs that the procedure may not be done optimally are the following: (1) Procedure takes less than an hour to perform on the entire face, (2) You ask how many pulses are being used and they answer less than 300 pulses for the entire face.

I was amazed that even physicians who come in to see me as patients also fall for hype and con-maneuvers. I found out that a patient who is a physician, and I believe to be a fairly intelligent woman, made the decision to not do the Thermage treatment with me and decided to go to someone else based on the following reasoning: I told her honestly that patients may get better results by doing more than one Thermage treatment so that I recommend that patients consider doing a second treatment a few months after doing their first treatment of Thermage. I told her from my experience that patients can get better results by doing up to 2 treatments of Thermage a few months apart. She then consulted with another physician who told her that he guaranteed she would only have to do one treatment to get the best results. What was amazing was that she concluded from all of this that I was "forcing" patients to get 2 treatments whereas this other doctor was promising patients they'd only have to do one treatment. This made me almost go crazy because it made my head hurt so much thinking that this is what I get for being honest upfront with patients and clearly spelling out to them that there's nothing predictable and that it's best for them to be prepared that they may get better results if they do more than one treatment. I was astonished that she would fall for someone telling her that he could guarantee that she wouldn't need a 2nd treatment because I know from experience that no one on this earth could make that guarantee. Also, why didn't she realize that in the end, if she didn't have any results, then the other doctor would then reveal to her that she may have to do another treatment, and why would that leave her any worse off than me telling her upfront that that would be the case?

The worst part is that the other doctor actually charged more for the one treatment and she ended up getting no improvement and concluded that the treatment must not work. I have never had a single patient in my practice have no results with the Thermage treatment. I know for a fact that many other patients getting treatment from other practitioners often report having no results. I also felt maligned by this patient leaving my practice thinking that I was "forcing" people to have 2 treatments—I have it clearly stated in writing that a patient "may" desire having more than one treatment and it is their choice whether or not to have a 2nd treatment, but that I wanted people to know upfront that some people will get better results by having a 2nd treatment.

In the particular case of this patient, I know that she would have gotten a more thorough treatment in my practice and she would have paid less for that treatment. She actually would have seen some results instead of getting zero results as she did with the other physician. In addition, I had already informed her upfront that she may desire getting a 2nd treatment to get even better results. She was not "required" to get a 2nd treatment, I just wanted to help her establish realistic expectations and help her understand that results can be improved upon by doing multiple procedures. It was disingenuous of the other physician to purport to guarantee any results, especially to claim optimal results after one treatment when there has been absolutely no scientific evidence to back up that claim.

Physicians are not infallible and that's why they're susceptible to cons and deceptions as patients and even more susceptible to industry's false promises as practitioners. They often turn around and repeat these fallacies to their own patients, not knowing that they're being preyed upon by companies for their naiveté and ignorance. The worst practitioners are the ones who knowingly present fallacies to their patients just to make a quick buck. Patients eventually discover the truth but too late. Unscrupulous practitioners figure there will always be another sucker born every minute.

My philosophy in my practice is based on being honest and ethical with my patients. My business model is based on repeat customers. Compare this to other practitioners who run a mill that is based on volume and getting high volumes of people in and out and having a high turnover. These mills count on getting large numbers of people in and out, and count on always getting more new customers by placing lots of ads, lowballing prices, and making promises that they can't keep. They know they can sign up a lot more patients if they tell them what they want to hear rather than telling them the truth.

CHAPTER 9:

THE FUTURE FRONTIER

WHAT DOES THE FUTURE hold? Vending machines for Botox®
and fillers? Cosmetic Salons for your pets where they'll do you at the
same time? Home laser razors to treat any hair on your body in the privacy of your own home? Fat melting devices? For good or bad, technology and innovation are constantly changing the beauty and cosmetic
industry.

The cry for insurance companies to pay for complications arising
from badly performed cosmetic procedures entered upon by unsus-
pecting or worse, consciously reckless, consumers trying to save money,
will cause a drain of our already rapidly depleted health care dollars to
deal with potentially catastrophic and life-threatening consequences
resulting from outright disregard of medical standards and principles.
It will divert huge amounts of resources, funds, energy, and time towards solving a problem that really shouldn't have occurred to begin
with. This is a man-made disaster, one that can be controlled.

Do you think we should pay for the complications resulting from
patients going down to Mexico or South America to get cheap cos-

metic surgery from questionable practitioners? Should the American public have to finance the ill effects resulting from patients making bad decisions that are risky just to save money for a procedure that's elective to begin with? Financial responsibility is an individual burden to carry and we should all bear that burden. As long as there are hucksters and charlatans and con-artists willing to take advantage of people's naiveté and greed, then there need to be protective mechanisms to punish those who exploit others and also protections against having to fund the misbegotten reckless behavior of those who aren't intentionally meaning to do harm and those who are unable and unwilling to watch out for themselves.

Educating the public is the first step. Social responsibility needs to be taught first in families and schools, and needs to permeate the entire fabric of our society with politicians, leaders, and role models setting the example. Social responsibility is the basis for collectively working towards common solutions to problems. It is the concept that we are all responsible for problems and no one person is completely exempt from the solution. We need to see the problems as they affect society as a whole, and not just focus on the individual victims and perpetrators. Social responsibility is the ultimate goal to impress upon the American public. Proper rules and legislation to safeguard the public from the dangerous effects of improperly performed laser procedures need to be instituted, and more importantly, enforced by the various agencies assigned to do so. Public mandates governing proper laser usage need to be established, and proper registration of laser ownership need to be set up and tracked.

Some basic steps that need to take place on the state level are the establishment of safe laser protocols and procedures, who gets to use the lasers and under what conditions. There needs to be a state and national registry of laser ownership so that any individual could contact the local agency to access the laser registry and find out if the practitioner that you're about to let treat you is properly registered as a proper owner of the laser.

The problem doesn't just exist in the U.S. The rest of the developed world is also experiencing similar problems with nonphysicians practicing laser surgery and medicine. In fact, conditions are probably considerably worse in other countries..

"Rogue plastic surgery clinics to be named" September 81, 2005. Quoting the British Association of Aesthetic Plastic Surgeons during a recent crackdown of illegal Botox activities, "Plastic surgery clinics that lure patients in with the promise of cheap deals and quick "lunch-hour" surgery will be named and shamed this week...treatments such as breast reduction and even Botox injections are being "trivialized" by cowboy businesses eager to cash in on the plastic surgery boom." The president of the BAAPS warned that the industry needed to "cool down". "We are increasingly concerned that frantic commercialization...is pulling surgical practice and medical decision-making into a marketplace frenzy," said Mr. Searle, a consultant plastic surgeon. Younger people and the elderly on budgets are especially susceptible to aggressive and unethical marketing practices.

The promise of cheap deals and quick "lunch-hour" surgery, and those who offer loyalty cards and discount vouchers to encourage men and women to undergo costly and often unnecessary treatment are rampant. According to an article appearing in the Wall Street Journal on January 3, 2006, there are more than 1500 medical spas in the U.S., up from a dozen or fewer five years ago. Many medi-spa owners try to sell their business within a short period of time, discovering that running a medi-spa is more complicated than imagined and also the profit margins are very narrow. Very few medi-spas manage to be financially viable. Besides potentially causing great physical harm to patients by improperly performing procedures, these spas cause many patients to invest money in prepaid packages that are never honored. Due to their financial instability, they often close down before performing the treatments.

Most of the dangers and problems with nonphysicians practicing medicine are immediately obvious. Corporations are not licensed to practice medicine and most states clearly define it as illegal for them to either partner with or control physicians' decision-making abilities. Besides the blatant examples of scarring, burning, and disfigurement, other dangers lurk when nonphysicians or non-qualified physicians perform laser treatments. Only dermatologists are trained specifically to recognize and treat skin conditions. It is unreasonable to expect that anyone else could competently spot and treat appropriately melanoma and other skin cancers. Incidences of skin cancers being "treated" with lasers (because they were misdiagnosed as benign skin lesions) have been reported. Also because of the high variability of response that individuals have to any treatments, the ability to understand the science of the skin when treating with a laser is essential. Melding the ability and training of understanding the body's largest organ (the skin) with the skills and qualifications to operate a laser is quite rare. Having the knowledge on how to devise proper treatment parameters goes beyond even what dermatologists receive in their residency programs. Money has clouded the judgment of many and has made many risk the safety of their patients.

The slippery slope of illegal activity has started. It started with physicians who did not properly supervise procedures and followed with physicians who were not trained or qualified entering the field. Their lack of knowledge and training encourage nonphysician staff (who in many instances knew more about the procedures than the doctor) to believe that they were qualified to perform these same procedures on their own in the context of their own business. Unscrupulous manufacturers and carpet-bagging physicians pushed and promoted the business of "cosmetic" medicine to all who would listen. When competition and sales tightened, they hit the nonphysician market with total abandon—patient consequences and the law be damned. Nonphysicians, lured by a market that they previously thought off-limits rushed in without evaluating the ethical considerations. Many, knowing that they were already skirting proper conduct and violating legal guidelines, ventured into outright illegality in order to prosper. Case after case has come forward of people being victimized by the injections of dangerous, non-FDA approved substances, permanent scarring from botched treatments with lasers, crippling pain following substandard care, and in some instances death. All of this continues unabated with laissez-faire attitude of the governing medical boards, politicians, and professional societies.

Investing in companies that have business strategies to bolster sales by promoting the illegal practice of medicine are not sound investments. Investors should carefully scrutinize the business plans of the corporations they invest in and also pay close attention to any laws being broken. America cannot tolerate anymore Enron and Tyco fiascos. Corporate America has to learn that conducting business on the fringes is a bad way of doing business. Investors should insist that the companies they invest in are doing business on the up and up.

Unfortunately, there are too many investors looking for quick gains and like the aggressive strategies of companies that really push the legal and ethical barriers. On the one hand, it seems smart to invest in a company that is selling more lasers to salons and spas—their numbers speak for themselves. They will sell more lasers in a larger market. Other laser companies will actually be criticized by their shareholders about why they're not adopting the same strategies. Eventually, if there isn't proper enforcement of the laws, corporations that aren't bending the rules would be at a disadvantage and the pressure would be too great to follow the lead of the other companies that are "getting away with it" and profiting from taking such risks.

In order to have an even playing field, there needs to be constant monitoring and policing of the industry. The referees need to do their jobs. There needs to be adequate and consistent enforcement of the laws. The bad guys need to be punished so that the good guys have a reason to stay good. This is true on an individual level, truer still on the corporate level.

The laser industry also needs to reinvest in research and development and actually come up with new laser technology that actually takes us to the next level, instead of constantly reinventing the same old devices and just repackaging them to sell to larger and more naïve markets. Laser companies are getting fat and lazy off the easy sell—it's much easier to sell low-end devices that don't really do much of anything and lower the price and sell higher volumes to nonphysicians. And since they see the market is so much bigger for salons and spas as opposed to selling to only physicians, the impetus and priority is to produce more products for that market, rather than trying to engineer more effective lasers that would require more skill and training to use. It has been the case with lasers that the more effective lasers are also more capable of causing damage, so a lot more training and skill are required to use those lasers. They've "dummied" down the laser devices to make them "safer". Unfortunately, lower power devices may be safer but they're also less effective.

Eventually the public is going to wake up and find out that the Emperor has no clothes. The heavy promotion of low powered devices aimed at saturating the salon and spa industry to get high volumes of customers paying low prices for treatments that basically do nothing will eventually result in consumer fatigue and mistrust. They will eventually discover that their money is disappearing but nothing else is. The promises of younger and more beautiful skin will become a hollow one. Consumers will start to think that none of these treatments work. That would be unfortunate because there are many laser treatments that are very effective and can do wonders for turning back the clock and beautifying the skin. A true laser expert can make you look 10 to 20 years younger and help correct and eradicate a myriad of problems. It truly is possible in this day and age to have a brand new face and new skin. It's unnecessary to have to live with something that nature gave you that makes you miserable. We have the ability to change things. And it is possible to do this safely and effectively. But you have to start by seeking the proper information. Lasers are only half of the equation—remember that the laser is only as good as the person operating it. The laser is nothing without the artist who wields it in their hands. It is the skill of the laser expert that will help you achieve the best results—not the laser by itself.

Laser companies cannot survive by catering to a handful of laser experts. They need to make procedures reproducible and in doing so, take the most essential ingredient out of the laser treatment, which is the physician's ability to extract subtle nuances out of the laser and customize it to fit each individual's needs. The science of laser surgery is one that can be taught to everyone, the art is something only a few can master. A true laser expert can apply their knowledge and skills to any new laser and help enhance and optimize the laser's capabilities even far beyond what its engineers had imagined. They can only do this because of their mastery of the physics and physiology behind laser technology and the clinical application and interaction of lasers with skin.

A good laser company that is interested in long-term growth would welcome the comments of a laser clinician/researcher no matter how critical or negative they may be, because only a laser expert who is actively engaged in the treatment of patients on a daily basis using their requisite knowledge of lasers and skin interaction and possesses the necessary clinical acumen that can only be achieved by being the ultimate end-user of the device can truly have their hands on the pulse of the industry—their opinion is vital for a laser company to be able to develop new and better devices and to continually improve upon existing technology. Companies interested only in short-term profit gains and not long-term growth constantly suppress the objective opinions of candid laser experts, not wanting to hear negative feedback and only wanting to push forward hype in order to sell more devices. They will, in fact, try to discredit those physicians who do not support their products, regardless of what the objective scientific evidence supports.

Many laser companies have come and gone. The ones that will remain standing are those that structure their business on sound engineering, research, and development. They produce lasers that really do something. They put more money and resources into product development than in marketing and advertising. They have a corporate philosophy which is based on building relationships, recruiting and retaining talented individuals, investing in new technology and research, diversifying, networking, building extensive distribution centers, nurturing forward vision, and promoting ethics and integrity.

Lasers are such a new industry that the laws and regulatory agencies have not been able to keep up with its huge growth. And because it is the "Wild Wild West" and "anything goes", it is paramount for consumers to be aware of the perils and watch out for themselves.

What can the public do to protect themselves?

1. Only go to a facility run by a physician **board-certified in dermatology** where the physician is on-site and evaluates you before any procedure is performed and will make the decisions regarding treatment.

   You can find out if a dermatologist (or any other physician) is board-certified by contacting the American Board of Medical Specialties. Their website is:

   www.abms.org

   (One caveat: you have to register with the site to get a password.)

The American Academy of Dermatology and the American Society for Dermatologic Surgery are excellent resources for finding information on qualified dermatologists. The following online sites provide a directory of dermatologists:

www.asds-net.org
www.aad.org

One major caveat is that the AAD and ASDS, although highly regarded organizations, do not list whether a dermatologist is board-certified. But they're at least a good starting point.

2. Ask questions about the physician's qualifications—do not accept that the physician is "trained in treating the skin" or that they are a "skin expert". If they do not clearly state and put in writing that they are a board-certified dermatologist, then you can assume that they are not!

3. Ask about the physician's training in lasers. Find out if they are a "dabbler" or a trained laser practitioner specializing in lasers. Evidence of a dabbler would be doing lasers once a week or twice a month, renting lasers, owning only one laser and claiming it does everything, etc. A physician specializing in lasers would own many lasers and be doing many laser procedures everyday.

4. The ideal physician to perform laser treatments is a **board-certified dermatologist** who has **fellowship training** in lasers and cosmetic surgery.

The media has presented over the past few years an increasing number of stories of botched-up cosmetic surgery being performed by nonphysicians and mistakenly treated them as if they were anecdotal occasional cases. They are not anecdotal, they were signs of the impending tidal wave that was about to hit, and now it's a category 5.

As the number of complications mount, increasing numbers of people are cheated out of their hard-earned money, and more and more laser spa/salons and chains fold under leaving their investors broke, there's going to be increasing legal action that will force state and governmental agencies to crack down on the rapid proliferation of illegal laser salons. There will be increased legal activity and accountability foisted on laser companies which will have to reign in their aggressive marketing tactics. They will ultimately be held liable for selling lasers to nonphysicians and for the undesirable consequences that follow.

Most importantly, the consumer needs to stop expecting the government to step in and regulate and control everything. The consumer needs to be aware that even if there are well-established laws and guidelines governing proper practice of medicine and cosmetic laser surgery, there may not be adequate enforcement of the laws. So it's buyer beware! Seek to educate yourself. Knowledge will empower you and enable you to protect yourself from harm. Reading this book is a good first step. Congratulations for being a knowledge seeker.

Addendum:
Laws Regarding Laser Usage and Medical Practice Ownership

Laws vary from state to state. Here are the laws regarding laser usage and ownership in California (many states have similar laws):

1. Medical practices can only be owned and operated by physicians.

2. Physicians cannot partner with non-medically licensed people (ie: laypeople).

3. Non-medical corporations cannot own, operate or participate in medical practices.

4. Nurses cannot own a medical practice. They may only partner with a physician as a minority partner.

5. Only physicians can own lasers.

6. Lasers are prescriptive and restrictive devices. The use of lasers is considered the practice of medicine.

7. Aestheticians, cosmetologists, medical assistants (MA), licensed vocational nurses (LVN), electrologists, and laypersons cannot operate lasers.

8. Nurses cannot legally perform laser procedures or other medical procedures (i.e., Botox®, Collagen, Restylane® injections) in shopping malls, beauty salons, health spas, and private residences (regardless of supervision).

9. Doctors may advertise medical procedures under their own name or an approved ficitious business name. Nonphysicians cannot advertise as they cannot acquire an approved medical fictitious business name.

10. Nurses are required to only perform procedures under the direction of a physician who is knowledgeable of the procedures being performed.

11. It is illegal for a nurse to find a "sponsoring" physician.

If you find that anyone is breaking these laws, you should report them to the following agencies who are responsible for conducting an investigation:

Medical Board of California
1426 Howe Avenue, Suite 100
Sacramento, CA 95825-3236
(916) 263-2388
(800) 633-2322

Board of Registered Nursing
PO Box 944210
Sacramento, CA 94244-2100
(916) 322-3350

If the agencies investigate and confirm there has been illegal activity, the violators could be subject to a fine, professional reprimand, forfeiture of licensure, and criminal charges.

Appendix

Resources for information:

American Board of Medical Specialties
Website: www.abms.org
(One caveat: you have to register with the site to get a password)

American Academy of Dermatology
www.aad.org

American Society for Dermatologic Surgery
www.asds-net.org

American Medical Association:
Website: http://www.ama-assn.org/ (click on "DoctorFinder")

American Medical Association
515 N. State St.
Chicago, IL 60610
(800) 621-8335

The California Medical Board:
Website: http://www.medbd.ca.gov/Lookup.htm.
California Medical Board
1426 Howe Avenue, #54
Sacramento, CA 95825
Office #: (916) 263-2382
FAX #: (916) 263-2944

Every state has a similar state medical board in which you can request information on any doctor licensed to practice in that state.
Food and Drug Administration
www.fda.gov.

Printed in the United States
59438LVS00002B/493-675